Tales from the Clit

A Female Experience of Pornography

edited by Cherie Matrix

for Feminists Against Censorship

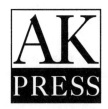

Tales From the Clit: A Female Experience of Pornography
ISBN 1-873176 09 0

Library of Congress Cataloguing-in-Publication Data
A catalogue record for this title is available from the Library of Congress.

British Library Cataloguing-in-Publication Data
A catalogue record for this title is available from the British Library.

Published by: AK Press   AK Press
P.O. Box 12766   P.O. Box 40682
Edinburgh, Scotland   San Francisco, CA
EH8 9YE   94140-0682

Front cover photograph by Grace Lau
Design and layout work donated by Freddie Baer.

This anthology is dedicated to my family — the tattooed, the devoted, the dead and gone as well as the living, but mostly to my cousin Avonna. Twenty-odd years, thousands of miles, and a world of flavour may have kept us apart, but we still both grew up to believe in the same thing: freedom, especially for women.
— Cherie Matrix

OTHER BOOKS FROM FEMINISTS AGAINST CENSORSHIP

Nudes, Prudes and Attitudes: Pornography and Censorship by Avedon Carol, from New Clarion Press, Cheltenham, 1994 ISBN 1 873797 13 3
Bad Girls & Dirty Pictures: The Challenge to Reclaim Feminism edited by A. Assiter & A. Carol, Pluto Press, London & Boulder, 1993 ISBN 0 7453 0524 5
Sex Exposed: Sexuality and the Pornography Debate edited by Lynne Segal & Mary McIntosh, Virago Press Ltd., London, 1992 ISBN 1 85381 385 0
Pornography and Feminism: The Case Against Censorship by Feminists Against Censorship, edited by Gillian Rodgerson & Elizabeth Wilson, Lawrence & Wishart 1991 ISBN 0 85315 742 1

Contents

Feminists Against Censorship's Preface _____ v
Avedon Carol and Cherie Matrix

Acknowledgements _____ ix

The Dirty Doctor: A (Brief) Career in Porno _____ 1
Arabella Melville

Indian "Purity" _____ 12
Meera Dharan

Lady O _____ 17
Deborah Ryder

A Deviant's Tale _____ 21
Jane Sweetman

XXX _____ 27
Christobel Mackenzie

Different Show _____ 32
Sue Raye

Pornography _____ 39
Helen Ryles

The Phantom in the Closet _____ 42
Rowan Green

Adventures in Pornoland _____ 46
Linzi Drew

Confessions of a Feminist Porn Teacher _____ 52
Jen Durbin

Access: All Areas _____ 50
Cherie Matrix

DIY Pornography _____ 66
Marcelle Perks

Erotique _____ 71
    Frances Scally

Pornography & Me _____ 76
    Anna Lynn Tercourse

The Best is Yet To Come_____ 83
    Annie Sprinkle

An Autopornography _____ 89
    Tuppy Owens

Blood Witch_____ 99
    Lucy Williams

Sexual Fantasy & Sexual Politics _____ 103
    Nettie Pollard

Pansexual _____ 107
    Val Langmuir

Self Portrait _____ 112
    Georgina Haynes

Body Parts _____ 116
    Avedon Carol

PORNUTOPIA _____ 121
    Lesley Ann Sharrock

NO NO YES_____ 126
    Caroline Bottomley

I Would . . . _____ 131
    Marisa Carr

The Scarlet Harlot _____ 134
    Carol Leigh

The Four Foot Phallus _____ 140
    Carol Queen

Preface

Imagine spending your whole life being told what you like and what you feel — and *knowing* that it isn't true. Doesn't take much imagination, does it? It's an experience we all go through. But until the late 1960s, women were expected to listen to what men told us about what all women felt, without replying. If we disagreed, there was something wrong with us, anyway. So women had consciousness-raising groups to talk about what we *really* felt. And now, women who call themselves feminists are trying to tell us that we all hate pornography, that no woman likes it, and that every woman wants to see it "off the shelf".

Feminists Against Censorship (FAC) was formed in April 1989 in response to other women who were claiming they could represent us all with this stereotype. We have spoken and written at some length now about the anti-pornography analysis, the research claims, the willingness to trust the state with decisions on what we should be able to see and say, and the misrepresentations that purport to support that claim. In *Tales From the Clitoris*, our fifth book, we have chosen to discuss our own, personal experiences of pornography. Strange as it may seem, precious little has been published in mainstream feminism from this perspective, particularly in Britain.

The political campaigning by anti-porn feminists has made it harder for women to produce their own sexual materials. It provides an excuse for the police to raid any shop, or seize any publication, that doesn't look like conventional, mainstream porn — "top shelf" material. This can leave British buyers with no legal choice but the uninspiring (and sometimes sexist) pornographic media that is made for men and usually by men. Images of intercourse, erections, genital contact and anything imaginative or mutual go by the boards when we are reduced to little more than pin-ups and strip-tease with no substance.

Some feminists in this book do enjoy this stereotypical male heterosexual porn. However, women have varied tastes and there aren't enough products on the market to quench our feminine thirst. And just why *is* the erect penis taboo in Britain?

Oddly, though, many anti-porn women in the United Kingdom do not realize that it is the law and the cops, and not something inherent in pornography or even in men's tastes, that makes British pornography so one-sided. They say they "don't like pornography" because there is nothing here to like — anything that is likely to appeal to women is likely to invite police raids or nondistribution by the major distributors. Women and sexual minorities who attempt independent production are the first real victims of anti-porn campaigns. And, as Arabella Melville shows within, the mainstream men's magazine producers like it that way — you might say Campaign Against Pornography keeps them in business.

Tales from the Clitoris' principal criticism of pornography itself is that most of it is about sex on men's terms. Until recently, almost all porn was aimed at men and even today much porn still is. Mainstream porn really excludes anyone who does not fit in with inviting, young stereotypes. However, we can't forget that this is true throughout most forms of media. Softcore pornography aimed at men plays it safe, by not showing erections or real sex, so that it can continue to be published, distributed, and sold.

Hardcore — that is, explicit material — is not legal in Britain's porn industry. Hardcore porn shows a variety of physical types, and as it tends to show people together, emphasizes that women can be assertive and in control, and not just young and passive blue-eyed blondes. One of our contributors, Jen Durbin from San Francisco, has studied the reality of hardcore porn in close-up, from a feminist perspective. Her experience in particular may be illuminating to those who fear having fewer restrictions on explicit sexual images.

Some feminists in this book enjoy fantasies and depictions of dominance and submission. These fantasies are rejected by many other feminists. Both lesbian and sub/dom porn are highly censored and publishers find it hard to get distributed. However, we all need to discuss our fantasies to help us understand the wide possibilities of female desire. Pornography has helped some feminists in this book to define themselves as sexual beings. Depictions of all types of women having all types of sex helps to clear away the mysteries surrounding female sexuality.

As well as criticizing the unbalanced maleness of porn, feminists are demanding a stronger position in the production of sexual imagery. Because of the lack of pornography for women, many of us have had to turn to other mediums for our arousal: inventing collages of stimulation from what sexual, and sometimes nonsexual, matter is available to us. Feminists want to see their fantasies on screen and read their desires in widely available magazines. The largest portion of essays in *Tales from the Clitoris* are from women who have never worked or had anything to do with the sex industry save their complete anticensorship stance. However, some feminists in this book have founded their own companies to produce and/or distribute feminist porn. Others supply stories and pose for various types of arousing material.

We want to emphasize the importance of publishing, as often as possible, the views of women who are more intimately involved with the sex industry — such as Linzi Drew — as well as of those who enjoy porn, since their voices are suppressed by the anti-porn movement and not given much credence by mainstream media people. Anti-porn women simply dismiss out of hand the testimony of women who disagree with them — if you aren't talking about how terrible pornography is, they don't want to hear it (and they may even accuse you of lying). But the media's approach isn't much better — women in the industry, no matter how bright and articulate, are treated as bimbos at best — purely a laughing matter. As feminists, we believe these women should be allowed to speak for themselves.

In sexist society, much of media, including pornography, is bound to contain sexism. Yet in this book, women from around the world, in all different circumstances, have found something positive to say about sexual imagery.

Pornography is one of the ways women in *Tales from the Clitoris* want to explore and evolve their sexuality. Many of the essays in this book elaborate on the way porn has helped women to see themselves as sexual beings, not victims, and empowered them to discuss desire. Other authors recount how, when growing up, most of their understanding of sex came from softcore magazines. FAC regrets that we all did not have a wider range of sex education material to learn from, and we do not want there to be even less of it for children growing up now.

Women especially need more sexual imagery, not more repression. Only through freedom from the guilt that we as women feel about our bodies can we become desirable to ourselves, not feeling as though we are "sluts" or "slags" for being sensual.

And let's remember that women's liberation is about opening possibilities for women. Pornography represents one of those possibilities — we should never participate in trying to shut it down.

Editor's Acknowledgments

I am appreciative of the dedication towards anticensorship that all of the women involved in this book have shown, especially Avedon Carol for endless consulting on her various expertise and pretty much doing everything short of coediting the whole book. Val Langmuir registers preferential applause for being the first person to see the book whole — then, take it home and proofread it for me. Particular thanks to Tuppy Owens who came up with the main concept of this book and, through her endless pestering of both business and personal contacts, found many of the pieces for *Tales*.

Feminists Against Censorship member Grace Lau donated the image for the cover and I feel it stands up on its own as a brilliant piece against censorship.

Special and personal thanks to photographer Della Grace whose work is not represented in *Tales From the Clitoris* due to unfortunate clashes. However, her interest in the project at a time when I was feeling that it would never end was very encouraging and gave me the drive I needed to complete the book.

I am grateful to Feminists Against Censorship for allowing me to edit *Tales From the Clitoris* on their behalf. They are an outstanding collective and I would like to spend more time just socializing with them; yet, unfortunately, we always have too much work to do.

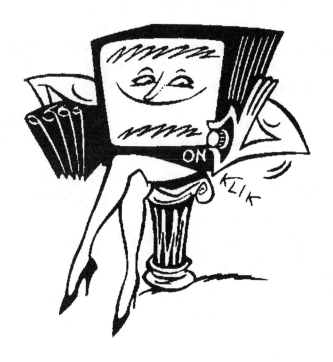

Other books have been written from the position of the hymen, but I write from the position of the clitoris.

— *Shannon Bell*

Arabella Melville is a writer and has published over a dozen books including Cured To Death: The Effects of Prescription Drugs, Natural Hormone Health, *and* Light My Fire. *Born in 1948 near Cheshire in England, her family tended to move around a lot. Consequently, Melville never felt part of any community. She has lived on boats, in caravans, flats and houses, in the city and in the country; mainly in England and Wales, but also in Canada, USA, Holland, and France.*

The Dirty Doctor: A (Brief) Career in Porno[1]

by Arabella Melville

I slid into porno in 1974 in the naive, passive way that I used to slip into most things at that time. I had few preconceptions; I was very innocent, and anyway, I saw myself as a scientist who would keep an open mind about things until I had evidence on which to base my conclusions.

After eight years at university, collecting degrees and learning about neurochemistry, animal behaviour and how to succeed in the scientific community, I gave up my academic career. It was a time of inner turmoil. All my plans for the future had been blown away by a moral crisis centred around the use of animals in scientific research.

Like most scientists, I had been hardened by my training to the suffering of laboratory animals. But my defenses were not sufficient to blind me to the pointless cruelty of a series of experiments that I watched in the physiology laboratories of Iowa University. I vowed that I would never do anything like them, but found I could not draw any logically defensible line between torturing decorticate rabbits in Iowa and what I had

---

[1] "The Dirty Doctor" was the title given to me by the *News of the World*, a daily English newspaper in 1975.

been doing elsewhere, like keeping hungry, thirsty or drugged rats in small cages.

At this point, I found I was unemployable. Refusing to do what I was trained to do, I discovered that nobody wanted to employ a woman with an irrelevant Ph.D. and no experience of anything but academic life.

That was when I started to take my clothes off for photographers. I had spurned the "respectable" world: now I was forced to learn to survive somewhere else. I can't say I enjoyed it, nor that I liked most of the products of my exposure. But my libertarian inclinations, combined with curiosity and my inability to find any other way to earn a living, led me deeper into that strange and seedy world.

I worked in grubby basement studios, where amateur photographers would book an hour with a nude model, and snap her in their favourite poses. Some came equipped with ropes to tie the model to a chair. These, ironically, were the mildest of men; I never felt threatened. Others wanted me to dress up as a schoolgirl. Some kept a furtive hand in a trouser pocket, wanking furiously while the other hand fiddled with the camera lens. I didn't care. I was only there for the money, and what they wanted to do was up to them so long as they didn't touch me.

I posed for girlie magazines, one of those grinning women in stockings and suspenders. I arched my back, stuck my tits and bum out and pretended to look inviting, but never took it seriously. Despite the growing disgust expressed by some members of the women's movement, I couldn't see any harm in men drooling over pictures like these. It struck me as rather sad that so many seemed to need this substitute for reality, even sadder that some were clearly so scared of reality that an inert substitute was as much as they could handle.

But I knew this couldn't go on. I was searching for an identity, a future, a career. After a few months, I decided on my goal: I would be a writer. Then, my Ph.D. would be an advantage, not a hindrance. I had no idea what might be involved in becoming a writer but I felt confident I could do it. I just had to seize my opportunity when it came.

My first commission came from Gerald Kingsland, later to become famous as the foul-mouthed anti-hero of *Castaway*.[2] Gerald had been taking photographs of me for his magazine *Curious*.[3] I was to write something based on my own sexual experience.

That was fine by me. I had been going through a period of self-discovery and experimentation, trying — in the way that was fashionable at the time, though I didn't realize then how far I was a fashion victim — to liberate myself from my sexual hang-ups. I'd been proving, in the most pleasurable way, how many of my mother's beliefs were nonsense: like, women can't enjoy sex without love, and no man will respect a woman who sleeps around. I'd read Germaine Greer and the growing literature of the feminist movement, spent many hours in consciousness-raising groups, and gone a long way towards replacing implanted embarrassment and shame with self-respect.

I had plenty to say. It was a time of such rapid change that anybody who actively sought experiences, and thought about them, had plenty to say. And I had degrees in psychology which, although actually irrelevant to real life and the understanding of it, allowed me to present myself as more than merely a moderately pretty face and bum.

I don't remember whether that piece was published. I certainly never got paid for it. What did happen was that through Gerald I met Colin Johnson, whose company distributed *Curious*. Colin and I became lovers. Twenty years on, we are still partners, still in love.

---

[2] Gerald Kingsland is best known for his practice of setting off for desert islands with young women. One of these was Lucy Irving, whose international bestseller *Castaway* (1983) was made into a film starring Oliver Reed.

[3] *Curious* was an unusually honest sex magazine published in London by Gerald Kingsland in the early 1970s.

Colin introduced me to *Suck*. This was the Real Thing: a sex paper that baulked at nothing, that included not only the raunchiest sex in words and pictures, but also had some of the most emotional and intimate writing I'd ever seen. Reading *Suck* was a revelation. It was erotic, it turned me on, it amazed and delighted me. Through its pages I met real people, writing about real sex and about fantasy but distinguishing between the two, not passing the latter off as the former. It was beautiful, too: designed by artist Willem de Ridder, edited by anarchist poet William Levy, it was so different from the tawdry girlie magazines for which I'd been posing, it reflected a different world.

In *Suck*, sex wasn't guilt-ridden, sexist, limited and somehow grubby. It involved the whole body, emotions and thought, and the whole spectrum of feeling, from pain to glorious ecstasy. Produced in Amsterdam, it was banned in Britain; the difference between *Suck* and British magazines reflected the gulf between Dutch and British attitudes to sex, censorship and personal freedom. Out of principle, Colin imported a few hundred copies to sell inconspicuously through a limited number of shops in London.

One of Colin's desires was to publish a new, wild sex magazine, a cross between *Suck*, *Oz*[4] and *Forum*. A passionate anarchist, he wanted to confront the Obscene Publications Act and all the other forms of censorship in Britain. We decided to work on it as a team. I agreed to take care of the words while he would do the visual stuff — pictures and layout. So a small publishing company was set up on the first floor of his Leicestershire warehouse, and I discovered the world of porno.

---

[4] *Oz* was the best-known publication of London's underground/alternative press during the late 1960s. It was very innovative in both style and content, and became known as much for its amazing artwork and use of colour as for its articles. *Oz* caused outrage because of its attitude to illegal drugs and its attacks on the hypocrisy of society. In a famous trial in 1971, the *Schoolkids* issue was found to be obscene; but the editors were acquitted on appeal.

Some of it excited me; some astonished me; much was uninteresting; some disturbing. I was annoyed by the fact that very little I saw or read was produced for women, or from a female perspective. The pervasive assumption was that only men were interested in erotica; women were merely objects of male desire. I was particularly enraged when an Oxford-educated magazine distributor, on being introduced to me, turned to Colin saying, "What's she good for, apart from the obvious?"

Our magazine was called *Libertine*, a title given to us by Gerald Kingsland. *Libertine* was funny and serious, campaigning and entertaining, unsophisticated in its appearance, yet a product of deep thought and discussion. I tried — not entirely successfully — to eliminate sexism from its pages and to make it equally interesting to both men and women. This proved difficult because the material available to us was almost always produced by men, for men, and I couldn't write the whole magazine myself. Nevertheless, a survey revealed that about a third of our readers were women.

As the magazine became established, my post bag grew. In my role as editor, I came over as a real person and the readers appreciated our honesty. While many expressed delight at our novel approach, others would write to me about their problems. I was shocked at the amount of misery I encountered. So many sad men: homosexuals, imprisoned for their sexual preferences; rejected transvestites; people with sexual and marital problems. I'd never realized there were so many anxious, guilty, oppressed and frightened people.

I wanted to help. I felt that liberation from sexual guilt was an important cause, for which I was a missionary: I saw sexual repression as a source of violence, self-loathing and despair. I wanted everyone to enjoy sex as I did. I wanted to change social attitudes, to change British society from one which condemned sex as dirty to one where sexual delight could be celebrated. The magazine was our vehicle for challenging established attitudes.

We knew that we would, in due course, find ourselves confronting the forces that exist to keep Britain miserable. "There is no reference to fun in any Act of Parliament," the judge had said at the trial of *Oz* a few years before. We understood that portraying sex as fun, attacking censorship and demanding only that there should be informed consent for any sexual act, would infuriate the legal and moral establishment.

Within a year, the Obscene Publications Squad turned up to raid us. We had a book shop in Leicester at the time; I was alone behind the counter when the police came in. They locked the outer doors, informed me that they had a warrant, and began to search and confiscate whatever they regarded as evidence that we were publishing obscene material.

I trembled; I felt sick; I was terrified. But I was convinced that what we had been doing was morally correct; that informing people about sexuality was socially beneficial; and that censorship was abhorrent. So I knew I must stand firm and take this fight as far as it would go. If I ended up in prison, so be it.

Colin, true to his nature, made things as awkward as possible for the police when they emptied his warehouse. They were there for sixteen hours, still carting magazines into police vans in the early hours of the next morning. They took thousands of copies of *Oz*, *Curious*, girlie magazines like *Fiesta*, and of course, *Libertine*. Personal letters, photographs and address files went too, never to be returned.

We thought we would be unable to continue publishing, but an angel arrived in the shape of Jill Tweedie. Her *Guardian* [5] feature about me and *Libertine* brought help from a wide range of sources: small sums of money from supporters; articles, poems, stories and photographs from new and talented contributors; and an offer of typesetting and other facilities from a gay publisher who had also been raided that summer.

---

[5] Daily paper published in the UK.

Then we confronted the obstacle race of the legal system. We were charged under Section 2 of the Obscene Publications Act, which meant a Crown Court trial and the threat of up to three years in prison plus unlimited fines on each of three counts, and we knew our only hope of winning the case lay in a brilliant defense.

Predictably, perhaps, we were refused legal aid, but we refused to accept the decision. Colin and I occupied the local court office, a dark basement under Leicester Town Hall, demanding to know the rules they were supposed to follow. The clerk tried to fob us off but Colin was adamant: we would not move until she gave us something on paper. Eventually, recognizing our determination, she disappeared into the bowels of the building to confer, returning with the information we needed.

With that ammunition we were able to overturn the decision and get legal aid for a solicitor. We chose David Offenbach, who had defended *Oz*; he got us money for a junior barrister, which was enough to engage the most brilliant team we could ever have hoped for: John Mortimer and Geoffrey Robertson.

The legal machinations lumbered on for eighteen months, a dreadfully long time to have the threat of prison and bankruptcy hanging over your head. The process itself punishes people: once accused, you are caught up in a system which induces stress, costs money, and takes up a staggering amount of time. The seizure of stock caused cash-flow problems which would have crippled a less healthy business than Colin's.

During this period, we were summoned to Scotland Yard to answer for ourselves. The formal interview was over quickly, with a series of "No comments" in response to every question after name and address. But the informal interview was most enlightening.

The police expressed surprise that I was clearly not the hard woman they expected me to be, and offered me the freedom to walk away, to have the charges dropped. I refused: this was an ideological battle and I was not about to back out. They suggested that we should stop publishing all our political stuff, and just sell lists of contact numbers for prostitutes and the like; that way, they assured us, we'd make plenty of money and they wouldn't bother us. "Wouldn't that be living off immoral earnings?" Colin queried. They didn't answer; but our lack of interest made it obvious to them that making money was not our primary aim.

Then the senior officer — second in command of Scotland Yard's Obscene Publications Squad — made a remark that astonished us with its perspicacity: "Don't you realize, if you succeeded in doing what you are trying to do with this magazine, you'd change the whole way of life in this country?" Exactly.

Finally we came to trial in February 1977. For a week, David Barker Q.C., Counsel for the Prosecution and the most boring barrister I've ever heard, sneered at our publications and accused us of trying to deprave and corrupt the public in general and children in particular. His speeches were so tedious that the press bench would empty every time he stood up. In reply, Mortimer and Robertson produced a wonderful firework display of wit and logic that often had the court roaring with laughter as they pointed out the absurdity of the charges against us. The local hack lovingly reported the defense case in each day's issue of the *Leicester Mercury* to refresh the memory of the jurors; most of the prosecution case went unrecorded in the press, too dull to be worth repeating.

The trial had several unique features. One was our choice of jury. Convention held that women should be rejected from the jury of such cases, but we would not discriminate on the basis of sex. Ours was the first mixed jury in an obscenity trial. Another was our range of witnesses. It included feminists and ordinary readers of the magazine, there to tell the jury they didn't feel they'd been depraved or corrupted. A third was our defense strategy. We argued that our magazine was "in the interests of learning": that it educated its readers about sexuality.

Although I quaked in the dock as we waited for the verdict, I could not believe the jury would find us guilty. And indeed they did not; the decision was unanimous, and we were free.

Colin thanked the knot of women from the jury afterwards. One responded in broad Leicester, "It were a load of old rubbish, weren't it, me duck?" I hope she was referring to the trial, not our magazine!

After the trial, we celebrated. We were free from the attentions of the Obscene Publications Squad; having failed once, in full public view (for we had organized a great deal of press coverage for the farce of our trial) we felt confident they would not readily go for us again. In fact, we heard some months later that another publisher — not a rival, for there were no others like us, but one which felt threatened by our determination to attack censorship — tried to get us raided. At that time, a thousand pounds paid to the right police officers in London would buy a raid; it was a well-known way of making life hard for competitors. But the Squad would not move against us. Too much trouble.

We were going all-out to create publications which would blow the Obscene Publications Act away. We realized we'd have to fight another trial, but we were willing to face that. We were planning to be seriously educational this time: revealing everything about sex in both pictures and words, exposing the plumbing, as we called it, so that we could at last move on from the ridiculous British obsession with anatomy to the far more difficult area of emotion.

But our troubles were not over. The girlie magazine trade saw us as uncontrollable, dangerous. They make money by trading on dissatisfaction; people who buy such magazines are constantly buying more in the hope of seeing a little more, searching always for the most explicit of a very uniform range of publications. If the readers could get what they wanted, they would buy fewer magazines; the collapse of the trade in Denmark had proved that. After a brief boom in sales when pornography was decriminalized, the Danish market had contracted to a small fraction of its earlier size. This was something which we would have welcomed, but which the others in the business were determined to prevent.

They intended to get rid of us. If the police would not or could not do the job, they would see to it themselves. We began to discover how the girlie trade planned to deal with us in early May 1977.

We were not invited to the meeting of magazine publishers, distributors and wholesalers in Charing Cross Hotel, London, but a friend passed the word and I was there. At that meeting (chaired, ironically, by David Offenbach), the girlie magazine trade expressed its intention of "putting its house in order" by establishing formal self-censorship. Mary Whitehouse, we love you. For the first time, they openly acknowledged their fear: that if things continued the way they were going, there would be "a Danish situation".

At that time, the British tits-and-bums soft porn trade was worth £30 million. That sort of money acts as a strong incentive to maintain the system that supports it. Censorship in this country is only indirectly directed by the law: the Obscene Publications Act defines illegal material as that which "tends to deprave and corrupt those who are likely to see it" — a charge which cannot be proved. There is no evidence, nor is there likely to be any evidence, that exposure to photographs of erect penises, for example, can deprave or corrupt anybody. When people who sell magazines refuse to take any that show such photographs, they are operating a system of self-censorship that has little to do with the law.

We could beat the police: there exist (if you can get them working for you) systems for doing so. But we couldn't beat the trade when it decided — for financial, not legal or ethical reasons — to establish a watertight system of censorship.

The means they chose was to prohibit any member of the trade from handling any sex magazine that did not carry a seal of approval awarded by a select committee chosen from their number. If anyone — from national distributor to corner newsagent — sold any magazine which failed this test, that person or company would not be allowed to handle any publication sold by any member of the group. That included many major magazines, not just girlie stuff. It meant, effectively, that anyone selling an unapproved publication would be put out of business. We put aside the magazine we'd been preparing, and produced an issue of *Libertine* designed specifically to conform with their requirements. It contained no contentious photographs, no dodgy cartoons, no reference to subjects like anal intercourse. We'd been in the trade long enough to know all the unwritten rules, though we had been breaking them for years.

As we anticipated, it wasn't approved. We knew that nothing we produced would ever pass. We were out of the publishing business.

Then Colin's company was bankrupted. All the stock he'd sold in May was returned, unopened, in August. Truck after truck rolled up to his warehouse in a single week, loaded with returns. And with every new pallet of untouched magazines there was a bill, for it had all been sent out on a sale-or-return basis.

It was, quite obviously, a carefully planned operation.

We lost everything we had. Even my car was snatched back by the hire purchase company. We left London with our sleeping bags on our backs and twenty quid borrowed from a friend, to struggle on social security in a caravan behind a chapel in Wales.

We survived, of course, to become writers and continue our sociopolitical agitation in different fields. But our porno phase was over.

Over, that is, until now. My latest book, I'm told, is pornographic, unsuitable for review in family newspapers. The censors of Wapping condemned *Light my Fire*[6] without trial. It's a book about sexual reality, about desire and emotion in long-term relationships: important issues, in my view. But the British establishment doesn't like reality. Acknowledging reality could, as the man said, change the whole way of life in our society.

---

[6] *Light My Fire* published by Michael Joseph, 1994; Fontana, 1995.

Meera Dharan is a 22 year-old British born Asian student with a long-term boyfriend (what a shame!!!). She lives in a residential middle class area in London. Dharan is fortunate enough to have parents who will not enforce an arranged marriage upon her. She is sexually active and guilt free. Dharan is not alone in her desires, as many Asian female friends have expressed the same sexual attitudes.

Indian "Purity"

Meera Dharan

My very existence as a British-born Indian woman appreciating the right to view and read pornography appears to have become a contradiction in terms. Originating from the land of the Kama Sutra provides little comfort for me, and absolutely no bearing in present day Indian society. I can imagine my parents' friends now, frowning and shaking their heads in solemn unison; " How could she bring such shame to her culture? She comes from a 'good family'. I can't understand what could make her write such filth." They will of course conclude that 'Western society' has somehow corrupted me. How strange it is for Indian society to make such condemnations, when our own art is so rich with deliberate, sensuous and voluptuous images.

'Pornography' is not a topic that enters the homes of most Indian families; however, one would be foolish not to draw inferences from deliberate silences. Sex is a taboo topic of conversation for the unmarried, especially so for Indian women.

Throughout my teens I had equated porn with unnecessary sexual excess. I assumed the women were short of money, forced into a degrading and humiliating profession. Those who produced porn, to me, were capitalizing on the declining morality of society. Perhaps the worst judgments I held were for those who bought porn — I labeled them as 'perverts' who were unable to cope with relationships of any kind. I had at this point not come into contact with any pornographic material. I know now that my views were based wholly upon a combination of my middle class and cultural background which together deemed porn as immoral — no questions asked.

University softened my harsh opinions. I was certain that porn could never appeal to me but understood why men might feel the need to relieve themselves; however distasteful the means, I concluded, porn was a necessary evil. Perhaps the turning point in my opinion was achieved while I was undertaking a project on pornography at university. I decided that to be objective I would need to see the 'unseeable'. I asked my boyfriend to purchase some so that I could make an informed decision on where I stood on censorship and porn. I was ready to feel shocked and vulnerable at the sight of women catering to men's pleasure. As I turned the pages of *Whitehouse*, *Playboy*, and *High Society* I was amazed at how little female submissiveness there was. If anything, I saw powerful women who were sexually aware, confident and in control — it was the rest of the media that portrayed women as the submissive sex, unable to cope without the 'capable man'. How could I have been so wrong? Ms. Catherine Itzin, you lied to me when you said that the pro-pornographers had a "callous disregard for the absence of women".[7] I saw no abuse as I sifted through pages of porn, all I saw was sexual interplay.

People have sex all the time, why does sex have to be so sacred all the time? Sometimes, some women would like to 'fuck' rather than 'make love'. My culture has placed enough guilt on me without the double burden of radical feminists telling me that I should be feeling disempowered by porn, when clearly I am not. Disempowerment to me means being turned down for a job for the colour of my skin, being told that I am incapable

---

[7] Itzen, C. *Pornography, Women, Violence and Civil Liberties*. Oxford University Press, 1992

because "I am only a woman". A woman having sex on film or on camera, being paid over three times as much as her male counterparts, looking sensual throughout, sounds more like empowerment than being rendered helpless. Why are we as women always expected to be the victims of male lust? The women I saw in the pornographic magazines seemed to have control of their sexuality and be in full control of their bodies.

My culture has little tolerance for those who do not conform to the submissive stereotypical female. Secret desires must remain so. I am silenced through fear of being ostracized and embarrassing my parents, who will be blamed for not exercising control over my thoughts and actions. How could I tell Indian society that I find the reading and viewing of sexually explicit material sexually exciting and it can help heighten pleasure in sexual interplay? As far as Asian circles are concerned I am still the submissive Indian virgin — at 22 years old, are they kidding?! The thought of an Indian woman enjoying pornography and sexual relations will prove too much, instantly making me the devil incarnate who will of course be the dangerous woman who mothers will want to hide their daughters and sons from, in fear that I will somehow corrupt them. No longer the dutiful and compliant daughter-in-law to be, but the woman with a mind of her own.

My 'virtue', 'honour' and 'moral fibre' will be placed under careful scrutiny. As old fashioned as these semantics appear, they are an accurate measure of Indian attitudes towards outward signs of sexuality. My interest in pornography extending beyond academic interest will be seen as an unnatural obsession. I feel condemned to hide my interest until I have reached the sanctity of independence, as it would provide me with the confidence and conviction to defend myself. Without independence I am forced into secrecy, my sexual soul is entombed by a restrictive and oppressive state. This schizophrenic existence of the 'good little Indian girl' on the one hand, and the liberated, morally confident woman on he other has been tearing me apart. This state of diaspora has caused me much pain and confusion, yet I have come to confront my lust and desires.

With all the virtues of Indian society, they may be unable to reconcile my opinions and ideas with that of their own. I have always been confused as to the correct Asian attitude towards porn. I still remember visiting Asian owned newsagents to find the top two shelves full of pornographic material. The greater irony is that if I were to purchase porn from an Indian newsagent that I would receive strong disapproving looks with with mutterings of immorality under his breath. Yet if they believe it is immoral, who is it that commits the greater crime: the person who purchases such 'evil' or the person who supplies and receives money from the sale of that 'evil'?

I am more than a prospective wife and child-bearer; my sexuality cannot be denied. Being the untouched sensuous virgin simply is not me. I enjoy watching porn, although if the truth be known, I wish there were better produced porn films and magazines. If it is not the Obscenity laws restricting porn, it is the lack of finance. Like my dislike of cheap films and cheap wine, I do not like cheap porn — although there is sometimes the occasional gem — but in the main I like good direction, production, lighting, acting, and plot from a porn film — I can ask for nothing more.

Why can no one recall the Gupta period in Indian history where sexuality was prevalent in art, until the thirteenth century when Islam became a powerful force in India? The banning of sexual representations of the human form in India ceased the production of sexual images dating from before the third millennium BC. Indian gods and goddesses are overtly sexual — especially Kali (goddess of destruction). Why are Indian people pretending the beautiful sexual images are not there, condemning those who then use it to explore their own sexuality; what went wrong?

My true sexual inclinations must be hidden. I have to fight the guilt placed so beautifully by Asian attitudes that always seem to bring 'the family honour' into every confrontational aspect of life. Because of my culture and a need for total honesty I have adopted a pseudonym. I feel very disheartened by my need to hide behind this veil of anonymity, but to survive in an Asian society a guise of purity is essential, as I am not prepared to find out the extent of Indian wrath.

Deborah Ryder is 47, although with her slim body and radiant com-
plexion she does not look it. Since she was very young, Ryder has been a
masochist. Her many published works include Half Dressed, She Obeyed
— a collection of erotic fiction representing the most powerful female
masochistic writing since Pat Califa's Macho Sluts.

Born in and still somewhat emotionally attached to Yorkshire, En-
gland, Ryder lived in London for some time, then migrated to Scotland
when multiple sclerosis forced her into giving up her career in a finance
company. Ryder is a member of the Outsiders — a club for people with
disabilities seeking partners. She believes that no one should have to
give up sex simply because they are disabled.

Lady O

Deborah Ryder

I am a masochistic woman; I write books on the subject of
submission/domination and have formed The LADY O Society
for submissive ladies. The need for such pressure-groups indi-
cates an unhealthy society. We, the few who know ourselves well
enough to accept and enjoy our own sexuality, are not obsessed
with sex; we enjoy it, in whatever form appeals to the individual.
Unfortunately this enjoyment is foreign to the repressed and
repressive majority.

At the root of the problem is the belief, common to most
governments, that they have the right to regulate the minds
and bodies of their citizens. Birth-control, fertilisation, abortion,
embryo research, harmless drugs, possession of defensive weap-
ons, holding a party, watching a video - you could be next in
line for the dawn-raid. Human rights mean nothing to the
British government, which advocates "Victorian values". In
Victorian times, the ruling class could have anything it wanted,
whether eleven-year-old virgins, pretty boys or bitches with

birches. The majority of the population lived in terrified respectability; the poor slept in the streets. Only one aspect has changed. Instead of "what will the neighbours think?", it is now "will the neighbours shop* us?"

So, no more excuses, justifications or rationalisations. We are the way we are because we enjoy it. The real reason why we cause such trepidation is because pleasure is - subconsciously if not consciously - regarded as wrong. Science has proven that no supernatural intervention was necessary in the world's beginning or to direct any event since then. But most people still need a psychological crutch. They need to believe in something because they are incapable of having faith in themselves. And, to perpetuate these belief-systems, they make rules; they forbid things. Sex, having always been a fairly widespread human activity, is an obvious target.

The TSNs (Thou-Shalt-Nots) have had it their own way for centuries. Things are not so different now, but there is a vitally significant, if small, transformation. When orthodoxy demands human sacrifice ("kill the unbeliever!"), there are a few who ask "Why?" The movement towards relaxation of censorship is inexorable. Always remember there will be setbacks. No-one wins all the battles. We shall win the war.

Being different does not damage the quality of anyone's life; and that should be the criterion. Sexuality disdains the "politically correct", which is just an updated version of "thou shalt not do anything enjoyable". We dare to enjoy; we dare to live. It is not surprising that the repressed majority envy and therefore hate us.

Mainly through economic factors — since economic factors are the prime motivation for anything concerning humans — the political situation is changing in many parts of the world. And because the new regime has not delivered Utopia, there has to be someone to blame. Those who are "different" are the

---

* UK slang for inform on

obvious target. If everyone was on the same wavelength, if everyone swung together, Utopia would be around the next corner, wouldn't it? But a few are spoiling it: the few who do not conform. The TSNs must put the blame on others because they cannot face the fact that they themselves bear a large part of the responsibility for the world's ills. The TSNs are the spiritual descendants of those who burned witches at the stake and forced Jews into gas chambers. But they wouldn't go so far nowadays, would they? Give them half a chance! Do you know how many people were murdered or seriously injured last year because their skin was the "wrong" colour or because they were gay? Several thousand in Europe alone. I do not have the facts and figures for other parts of the world, but why should they be different?

And consider another murderous machination by those whose religion is bigotry. Such pressure-groups are making objections (in some cases going so far as legal action) against sex-education for young people. Condoms must not be provided. Only the celibate deserve to avoid AIDS. In the long-term, this will backfire on the bigots, since they seek to deprive their own children of the knowledge that would keep them safe; and it is a fact of life that someone brought up in an overly-religious atmosphere will go out on the tiles as soon as he/she can. In the short term, this is just another maneuver by the forces of repression. We should be used to that.

Although we recognize this oppression, there is not much that we can do about it. Even activities in one's own bedroom are subject to the sanction of the law. There are a few pressure-groups to reassure each member of the persecuted minorities that he or she is not alone. Recently-formed, The LADY O Society intends to provide this reassurance for submissive ladies. We know the loneliness and isolation of this way of life. Whenever a new member says 'I thought I was the only one in the world', she reaffirms the need for such an organisation.

The feeble excuses for censorship are based on a claim to protect the weak. Who are these people who are so indecisive that they would be inflamed by seeing a video of a crime and would promptly go out and do it? If a person is going to rape and/or kill, the problem was in his head long before he read a book or saw a film. Yet we so often hear of the criminal who pleads "pornography drove me to it"*. He has been caught; his advisors are seeking to mitigate his sentence. Offer the Establishment a different target (a target which they never tire of attacking) and reduce the offender's culpability at the same time. Neither the accuser nor the accused is interested in the validity of the excuse because neither wants its fallacy exposed.

As a world-wide trend, it has been noted that the more liberal the society, the fewer the sex-crimes. This may be partly as a result of fewer sexual activities being criminalized, but it is mainly an indication of a generally healthier attitude to sex. Improve Law and Order — Legalize Pornography! The world is approaching the twenty-first century, but the law-makers of Britain and other countries have yet to emerge from the Dark Ages.

---

* Editor's note: For more information on this argument, please see another Feminists Against Censorship book, *Nudes, Prudes, and Attitudes* by Avedon Carol, Clarion Press 1994.

Jane Sweetman was born and raised in London, England. She has an Arts degree and has been writing sensual, yet rather selfish, prose for years. Sweetman has a tendency to over-indulge in anything that's damned, given half a chance!

A Deviant's Tale

Jane Sweetman

There seems to be as much disagreement about what constitutes pornography as there is about what constitutes obscenity, and probably for similar reasons, so I should begin by explaining that I tend to take a very simplistic approach to the whole issue: if an image depicts an aspect of sexuality or is intended to arouse sexual interest, it counts as pornography in my book, as someone somewhere will probably try to ban it. Perhaps I am confusing pornography with sexual imagery, but they seem to amount to pretty much the same thing and, since the word *pornography* can evoke some quite extraordinary value judgments, I am perfectly happy to swap words. Of course, that still leaves the distinction between hard core and soft core sexual imagery, but that is another matter. A lot of traditional pornography that decorates the top shelves of many newsagents is aimed at men and, when I was a young woman, I found it uninspiring to the point of alienation. Since it is only recently that I have found material that does interest me on the shelves, this tale is not so much about my experiences of pornography as a personal tale of pornographic substitution.

Even my mother would have approved of my earliest sexual fantasies. Each night, just before dropping off to sleep, I would masturbate to images of brightly wrapped Christmas presents, complete with ribbons and bows. I was not even slightly interested in what was within the wrappings — it was enough that all these presents were mine, waiting to be opened. At the time, of course, I did not know the name of the activity that accompanied these fantasies and I certainly had no concept of its sexual nature as, at that stage, my sexual awareness was limited to a rather clinical knowledge of the physical differences between boys and girls.

My mother was very protective of the sexual innocence of her children and, whenever we asked her about any matter relating to sex, she would tell us that we were too young to understand. Although she always promised to explain it all when we were older, it was a long time coming and, fed up with being fobbed-off in this way, I decided to find my own way through to this exciting and hidden adult world. On the pretext of having read all the books in the (rather small) local children's library, I gained my parents' permission to join the adult library and, once there, I avidly scoured the shelves for information.

The material in that library opened up a whole new world. I discovered, for example, that the word "prick" has more than one meaning and, at the same time, not to ask any family member the meaning of a word, since a good dictionary contains even the rudest words. In all innocence, I read out the words 'as stiff as pricks' to my brother, so that he could hear the context, which resulted in that particular novel being confiscated before I could read any further. Worse still, my mother then insisted on vetting all my library books and, until her enthusiasm for the task waned, I had to select books that I knew she would permit me to read. The trick then was to sneak off and replace them, later the same day, with something more to my own tastes. Of course, this made the whole thing much more exciting and much more shameful. Although my brother did, finally, explain the meaning of that troublesome word (once I had promised not to tell our parents) I still had to figure out what the sentence could possibly mean, and it took quite a while to read enough material to fit the pieces of that particular puzzle together.

Since I was denied access to information and material directly relating to sex in my early years, I started to create my own pornographic imagery from what I found within the pages of books and from the images projected through television. Sex is such a strong force that loss of innocence (as opposed to virginity) is a fact of life, and the important thing is whether it is replaced with understanding or ignorance. In my case the protective framework my mother constructed around me became a trap, made from ignorance and which formed a fertile breeding ground, creating sexual images from whatever material it could find. How and why one image becomes more sexually weighted than another is still a mystery to me. Some of my early favourites were war novels, written by people who had obviously been deeply disturbed by their wartime experiences, and this kind of material became a focus for my budding sexuality. Television became another such source, and I can vividly remember being fascinated by a scene in old Western film, where a cowboy was publicly flogging an Indian. At around the same time I also became fixated with war films depicting Nazi torturers and, horrified that I should find such foul acts sexually exciting, I tried to ban them from my thoughts. The transition from Christmas presents to torturers was a frightening one, but, for good or bad, these dark images were here to stay and I cannot help but wonder whether, had I been able to find some more direct sexual material during these years, I might have developed more along the lines that my parents had intended. Their attempts to protect my innocence, though well intended, did not work out quite as they might have expected.

I abhor real-life violence of any kind, but my tastes in fiction have always leaned towards violence and horror and, although this interest is not entirely sexual, there is a strong sexual element to it. When news broke of the activities of the first serial killers, I became seriously worried that I might already have taken the first steps on the road to this kind of madness. This fear spurred me to read as much as I could about the subject and, fortunately for me and for the rest of society, I lack many of the major characteristics of these compulsive murderers and have never felt any inclination to act out any of my darker, more violent fantasies.

The general lack of directness on matters of sex that I encountered, along with the normal problems of adolescence, generated strong feelings of frustration and aggression within me, and I gave vent to these, outside the home, in various ways — one of which was drawing rude pictures. I once took advantage of an inattentive teacher by spending a lesson drawing a picture of a naked man and woman, both of whom had wildly oversized sexual organs and, for good measure, little bubbles coming out of their mouths containing every rude word I could think of. Instead of destroying the picture, as I usually would, I left this one in a desk for the next lucky pupil to find. The act itself was accompanied by feelings of great hostility and resentment, followed immediately by shame and guilt.

I finally learned about the mechanics of sex at school, in a Biology class, when I was an adolescent. This went some way to correcting the rather murky, off-beat picture that I had managed to build up for myself, but for reasons best known to our elected sexual educationalist, there was no mention of the pleasure that can be generated within a sexual relationship. Indeed, the picture that we received was that, for humans, this act was something that was performed only within the bounds of marriage, and then only for the purposes of creating children. Since I had no intention of marrying or of having children, I found this a very unattractive proposition. I was persuaded, at a later date, to try some heavy petting, but I found it uninspiring, and it was not until my early twenties that I felt it was time to really take the plunge. Not unusually, I suspect, it was not all I had hoped it would be, but the sheer naughtiness of it was a great thrill. Unfortunately, I became stuck within the clinical boundaries of sex as laid down in that Biology class, and it was to be many years before I could fully appreciate the pleasures of sex, or before I discovered that there is pornographic material available which reflects and expands upon my own sexual preferences.

Surrounded by an atmosphere of secrecy, guilt and isolation throughout my sexual development, I would often worry about the nature of my private fantasies, and never spoke about them to anyone. I considered having treatment for my 'condition', but I was convinced that, if anyone ever found out how sick I really was, they would lock me up and throw away the key. Fortunate for me, then, was the discovery of the large and active S/M and fetish scene in recent years. This, with its dark and potent images of domination, rubber, leather, whips and bondage, has provided me with an ideal sexual outlet, supported by a wide range of specialist publications, all of which provides a more suitable setting for my fascination with images of power and pain than the cowboys and Indians of my youth. The freedom and acceptance that I have found within this environment has given me my first real taste of sexual freedom and fulfillment — a jaunty stride forward from my earlier days of non-orgasmic fornication.

Although this is all great fun, a more important benefit has been that, by allowing me to dispose of the twin burdens of isolation and guilt, it has added an entirely new dimension of passion and affection to my sex life. I feel as if the door to my sexuality has been opened and, for the first time in my life, I am able to enjoy sex as an exciting and fulfilling experience, sometimes spiced with fetish or S/M games and publications, sometimes not. Perhaps the most important element in all this is the discovery that there is a large sector of the population who share similar tastes and, although I have still not settled on one side or the other of the S/M fence (whether I am dominant or subservient depends entirely on my mood, or that of my husband), I am happy just to have the freedom to experiment.

From my own experience of growing up in a sexual desert, I feel certain that repressing or denying sexual interest is not a good way to deal with it. Children, in particular, are not well enough equipped to take charge of this area of their own development and, although I am not advocating their unsupervised exposure to explicit pornography, direct and open discussions on sexual matters with their parents or other adults can only be a good thing. We all need some acknowledgement of, and outlet for, this very strong and vital part of our natures, and surrounding sex and sexual imagery with an atmosphere of shame and secrecy can only be damaging. I am sure that my parents were trying their level best to protect me from corruptive influences throughout my childhood so that I could grow into a healthy adult, and I may well have still have centred upon images of power and pain whatever my background, but I cannot help but wonder whether this might have been a very different story had my parents given me the keys to open the doors to my own sexuality in a more informed way from the very beginning.

Christobel MacKenzie is an anarcha-feminist who has been quietly active for many years in international feminism, and is a member of the Anti-Sexism Campaign.

XXX

Christobel Mackenzie

When I was about 13, D.H. Lawrence's *Lady Chatterley's Lover* was acquitted of obscenity. Our tenants had bought a copy, and one Saturday morning I crept into their room and looked for the "dirty" bits. I felt guilty, but only really because I shouldn't have been in their room. The following year, I found Emile Zola's *Lolita* in my father's bedroom. I knew this was a scandalous book, so I had a look at it and enjoyed doing so.

When I was 14, boys secretly passed girlie pin-up magazines around the classroom. This was a male club that excluded women, and I remember thinking how different my body and projected personality were from the sort of women portrayed in those magazines. I couldn't compete, and I didn't really want to. I felt passionately that sexual relationships shouldn't be conducted on the grounds of what bodies looked like, but with the whole person. I still believe this up to a point, except that now I believe sexual attraction to bodies specifically can be positive and exciting. But I also find all bodies are attractive in their own way. I believe there are only unattractive personalities, not unattractive bodies.

In about 1968 I saw an ad in one of the "underground" magazines (either *International Times* or *Oz*) for pornography catalogues. I sent off for one and obviously got put on a mailing list, because (although I never bought anything) I received dozens of catalogues for porn books, magazines and films (this was before video). The catalogues included lesbian materials (made by men probably, using models) and gay male material, and some involving young people and also animals. I liked looking at the catalogues partly because they were taboo and they involved types of sexuality I didn't know about. I wanted to know more.

I went to work for the Arts Council of Great Britain when I was 19 and it was there I first met gays. I was also shown porn by staff members. I saw *Schoolkids* issue of *Oz*, which was prosecuted for Conspiracy to Corrupt Public Morals in 1971. This issue was entirely written by boys and girls still at school, and I remember seeing the original magazine at the news kiosk at Archway underground station. But I didn't buy it then because it had two black 'lesbians' on the cover, one with a vibrator, and I saw this as exploiting women. When I finally read the magazine (shown to me by someone at work), I remember tips on giving a blow-job using ice cubes in your mouth and blowing as well as sucking a penis, and the cartoon of children's character Rupert Bear fucking Gypsy Grannie. The fellatio tips I found intriguing, and the cartoon I saw as a blow against ageism — after all, why shouldn't an old woman be attractive to a boy? I know some Feminists saw it as a distressing sexualisaton of an innocent childhood story. I suppose, although I respect their feelings, I never saw childhood as innocent or non-sexual.

The first pornography I bought (1970) was a "marital aids" type book of various positions for sexual intercourse called *Making Love in Living Colour*. The couple was nude but obviously not really having intercourse. The book just showed about 50 positions. It was clinical but sort of exciting at the same time. I had never had a sexual partner and was hopeless on my own. At 22 I had never had a waking orgasm: although I used to get highly turned on, it never led anywhere.

Although my mother was informative about sex from an early age, I got all my subsequent information from pornography, and stories in the underground press, especially *International Times*, *Ink*,[8] *Oz*, and the American *Rolling Stone*.

---

[8] *Ink* was a left wing pro-gay underground paper.

I had my first sexual experience with an older man at work in 1971. The next year, I met a man at the *Oz* appeal and had sex with him on the night of the Miss World demonstration. The next year I started a relationship with a woman. Sex with a partner was easy and fulfilling. The years of frustration were gone. In the '70s there didn't seem to be any sexual materials made by or for lesbians — only really feeble porn aimed at men, showing bored-looking women with very long nails and lots of lipstick pretending to be ecstatic and not really doing very much together. At around this time I started buying the American gay literary magazine *Gay Sunshine*. This contained (amongst other materials) explicit sexual stories. I especially enjoyed the stories by men about how they had sex when boys, often with older partners. The fact that both (all) participants were male did not present a problem for my enjoyment. I have more recently learned that lots of women enjoy male gay porn.

The mid to late 1970s onward struck me as a rather sexless time politically. Lesbian and gay groups were being respectable and being state-funded by the GLC[9], etc. No one wanted to rock the boat. The Women's Liberation Movement was now "feminist" and seemed to be largely in disarray, concentrating on anti-sex campaigning against pornography, paedophilia and sex shops.

Then in 1988 something happened! Firstly, the government introduced Section 28, which outlawed "intentional promotion of homosexuality" by local authorities, and banned "teaching of homosexuality as a pretended family relationship". No one has been able to work out what on earth either of these things means. Lesbians and gays woke up and began to fight back. Out of this issue arose the lobbying group Stonewall, the civil disobedience direct action group OutRage!, and, indirectly,

---

[9] Editor's note: GLC (Greater London Council) was a governing body for the whole of the County. Disbanded by the Conservative Government in 1988.

the anarchist sexual liberationist Lesbian & Gay Freedom Movement[10]. Sexual politics wasn't dead.

The second thing to happen in 1988 was that Joan Nestle came over from America to promote her book *A Restricted Country*. This book had an enormous effect on my life, and I think on the lives of many other feminists and lesbians (and some gay men, too). *A Restricted Country* is a series of essays and fiction by a lesbian fem who came out in the late 1950s, about her life, politics, and fantasies. 1970s feminism had told us that Butch-Femme role playing was an overhang of heterosexism, and dildos (and indeed, penetrative sex of any kind) was a male myth about lesbians. To Joan Nestle, lesbian butches were the standard-bearers of gay liberation, and dildos were deeply erotic and female. Lesbianism wasn't just about politics, it was about sex!

On September 6th (my birthday) I went to Conway Hall at Red Lion Square in London with my lover and a close female friend to hear "Putting the Sex Back into Sexual Politics", a forum chaired by Mary McIntosh (later of Feminists Against Censorship), featuring, among others, Joan Nestle and anti-porn activist Suzanne Kappler. I remember Ms. Kappler saying that any kind of sexual representation in a sexist society was intrinsically oppressive to women and shouldn't be allowed. Joan Nestle said that as women, we own our own sexuality, and mustn't be dictated to by straight society, heterosexist men, or anti-sex feminists. There was a difference — an erotic difference (a power imbalance difference) — in wearing lipstick to conform to men's expectations of how women should be and wearing lipstick as a woman for women. Porn made by and for women was different from porn made by and for heterosexual men using women.

After that meeting, I somehow never felt things would be the same again. I directly trace the birth of Feminists Against

---

[10] LGFM is now called the Passion Brigade to encompass sexual diversity.

30

Censorship to this meeting. And indeed, a number of future members attended.

In 1989, *Coming to Power* (lesbian feminist writings on S/M) by the lesbian Samois collective was made available in this country. It was burnt in the streets by anti-sex feminists. To many of us, it was a revelation. We wanted to celebrate it, not to suppress it. Here was a book, like *A Restricted Country*, about women taking and using their power and sexuality for themselves and their lovers. Wasn't that one of the aims of the women's liberation movement?

Later that year, Feminists Against Censorship was born, and it seemed the natural place to be. . . .

Sue Raye went to an all-girl private school in Melbourne, Australia. The Methodist Ladies College recently contacted her for a twenty five year class reunion. As part of the reunion they were compiling a book and Raye was asked for a precis of her last twenty five years. Part of her precis went as follows:

1981   Personal Assistant to entrepreneur in entertainment industry.

*1982   Manager of **adult** video company, Electric Blue.*

1984   Transferred to Sydney as Product Manager for Electric Blue and Kideo Classics.

*1985   Formed own video distribution company, Video Ray Pty. Ltd., **specializing on adult videos and in particular erotica for women.***

1988   Became the distributor for the domestic market of Nina Ricci handbags.

*Fortunately, Raye did not attend the reunion, as when the book came out Methodist Ladies College had edited out **adult videos** and **erotica for women**. Raye was extremely angry and wrote them a letter asking how dare they edit her life. She received a reply advising that the College do not like to be seen endorsing past pupils' products. Interesting that they didn't delete the reference to Nina Ricci!*

Different Show

Sue Raye

Apart from the initial discovery as a toddler that boys and girls are different and the "you show me yours and I'll show you mine" routine that most young children engage in, my first recollection of "sex" was when as a girl of about ten years of age my parents would hide their copies of newspapers featuring a Page 3 girl. I couldn't understand why they were hiding them from me. Etched in my memory, however, is the picture of finding one such newspaper they'd inadvertently left within my reach on the top of the refrigerator (actually it wasn't really within my reach, I had to stand on a chair to retrieve it). I remember feeling very excited that I was about to look at something which I'd been told was naughty and forbidden. Upon finding a topless girl with the largest pair of tits I'd ever seen, I remember feeling a strange mixture of excitement and indefinable pleasure, a tingling throughout my whole body. I wonder whether what I was feeling was caused more from the pleasure of viewing forbidden fruit or from the actual image itself?

The rest of my teenage years were spent experimenting with sex and finally losing my virginity just after I turned seventeen. Pornography wasn't an issue during those years as censorship was still fairly strict in Australia and of course videos were a thing of the future. Besides, we were all having too much fun experimenting sexually with our friends to be bothered with any additional stimulus. It was the swinging sixties and we were all very free.

My first exposure to pornography happened in the early seventies when I was sharing a large flat in London with five English guys and another Australian girl. One of the guys was with the vice-squad and he brought home a porno movie they'd seized and screened it one night in the lounge-room of the flat. All the guys gathered around excitedly with myself and the other girl hanging around the edges of the room, not sure whether we should indeed be there infringing on this "male" domain. The movie commenced and the only feelings I can recall were ones of curiosity tinged with interest that such a big fuss was being made of viewing these images which were nothing more than two or three people having it off, albeit in close-up detail. I remember leaving after about ten minutes, mainly because I was bored with close up shots of male and female genitalia. If that was pornography then it certainly didn't turn me on.

I guess that first experience with pornography helped influence my views because many years later after a varied office career I was offered a job working with the original Australian licensee of the *Electric Blue* range of adult videos aimed at a male audience. Here was something totally different from the tacky images I recall seeing in the London flat: this material featured beautiful women in lavish surroundings, either pleasuring themselves or being pleasured by a handsome man or beautiful woman. This was definitely something I could relate to!

After working as manager of the *Electric Blue* office for a couple of years I then took on the Australasian distribution for myself and have now been involved with *Electric Blue* for more than twelve years. After running it for a while I realised something was missing ... female sexuality and female fantasies weren't being catered to. Whilst *Electric Blue* is very good quality, it is made by men with a male audience in mind and although women can and do enjoy it they can also be very bored with its focus on male gratification. I started looking around for video products we could include in our catalogue that I felt would appeal to women as well as men, and in my research read about Candida Royalle's *Femme* range of erotica for women and couples.

In addition to the *Electric Blue* and *Electric Fantasy* ranges we have now been distributing the *Femme* titles for over seven years and they have been very successful. It is interesting that sales in this country to the video rental libraries of the *Femme* product have been limited, which I put down to two reasons. Firstly, the majority of video buyers are male and as they have shelves full of adult material "down the back" of the shop catering to men, they don't see the necessity of having any product which caters to women's sexuality. Secondly, they don't believe, and to a certain extent they are right, that women will go into a video store and rent erotica for themselves. However, our experience shows that if you give women a chance to purchase via mail order, they will go for it. They can retain their anonymity which is important to them as we have yet to reach the stage where women in general will admit publicly that they enjoy watching erotica. I think this possibly stems from the poor image that has flown down over the years since video porn has been available when they were initially made purely as stimulus for men with the women's desires and needs totally ignored, where women were portrayed as men's play toys and no attention was paid to the women's sexual satisfaction. That's not to say that this type of product isn't still available: it is, but it's certainly not in my catalogue.

The overall quality of adult movies could certainly be improved upon if the producers were confident that larger production budgets would give them a significant return on their investment. Whilst the laws relating to the production and distribution of pornography are under constant threat of change it is understandable that producers are hesitant to spend a lot of money producing something that could be outlawed the next day.

After fourteen years in the adult industry I have probably viewed more adult videos than any other female in Australia and I do enjoy watching them although unfortunately it can sometimes become quite a chore, such as the times when I receive boxes full of tapes to preview. Unlike some of our competitors we don't include any titles in our catalogue that we haven't viewed and we also don't include any titles that have poor production values, poor acting or poor story-lines. Finding quality product is one of the hardest parts of the business and I live in hope that quality standards will improve.

The majority of adult movies are currently made by men and portray sex from a male point of view, catering to their own male fantasies. One aspect of these I find off-putting is the "money" shot at the end of each sex scene where the man (or men) ejaculates over the woman's face. It doesn't happen like this in real life and I find the portrayal of women enjoying men cumming over their faces as rather unrealistic. This is not what generally happens between consenting adults and I feel it tends to demean women when the screen shows a close-up of a woman supposedly enjoying having cum sprayed all over her face.

Being female and involved in the adult arena has sometimes resulted in some amusing situations. I recall going on a date with a guy one evening and on returning to my place I had to view a title we were having censorship problems with. I asked if he minded if I quickly checked out the video and he readily agreed as I don't believe he had ever seen any adult material and was obviously curious. Whilst I sat with pen and paper making notes he sat squirming in his chair and at the end asked me if I was embarrassed! Needless to say that was the last date I had with him! People's reactions are also very interesting when they find out what work I do. Some are fascinated and want to know all about it and others get embarrassed and quickly change the subject. I think a lot of people are shocked as I don't fit the typical stereotype of what someone working in the adult industry is like. They expect a big fat cigar-chomping bloke who is the epitome of sleaze and when they find a relatively attractive and smartly dressed woman who is successfully running a business involved with sex they just don't know how to handle it.

The hardest people to convince that what I do is quite normal are my parents, now both well into their 70s and unfortunately still retaining the moralistic and puritanical views of the majority of the older generation. I have tried on several occasions to explain that I am marketing a product which is legal and which depicts adults engaged in consensual non-violent erotic activity and provides thousands of couples with an additional stimulus to their sex lives and is an outlet for single, lonely or handicapped people who don't have a regular partner. Unfortunately my explanations fall on deaf ears as my parents have their firm views and aren't willing to accept that society has changed since they were young and that sexuality is no longer the taboo subject it used to be.

When I first started my business my parents were less than enthusiastic. I got the feeling they doubted my business ability but more importantly they didn't like the fact that their daughter was in the "sex" business. In their minds "nice girls" didn't flaunt their sexuality and I believe that's what they thought I was doing, even though I was only selling R rated videos. Growing up I'd always thought of my father as a "with it" type of guy, he was the senior airline pilot with the major domestic airline and had traveled extensively, both in Australia and overseas. He may have been "with it" as far as his mates were concerned but definitely not when it came to dealing with his daughter.

When the full impact of the AIDS epidemic hit around the mid 1980s the Australian adult industry decided that as a community service we would put together a safe sex trailer to be featured at the beginning of all X and R rated videos. The three minute trailer gave safe sex information and was explicit in that it showed how to put a condom on an erect penis. Under normal circumstances the Commonwealth Censorship Board would have given the trailer an X classification because it showed an erection. However because of its educational value and the fact that it would reach a far wider audience if also included on R rated titles the Board is to be applauded for giving the trailer an R classification.

The adult industry nominated me as the spokesperson for the launch of our safe sex campaign and I spoke on various radio and television programs including a high rating breakfast program on one of the major television networks. I was rather proud of what we'd done and phoned my parents to let them know I was appearing next morning on the breakfast program. Big mistake! A week went by without any contact from my parents and then I received a call from my father telling me that my mother wasn't well. When I asked what was wrong with her I was told "you're killing her . . . she collapsed in the kitchen and has been in bed, she can't face her friends because of what you've done and we want you to promise that you won't go on television again". Needless to say I was incredulous. I couldn't understand their attitude — why would they be upset because I was talking about *safe sex*? I would have understood their fears if they'd been upset because I was promoting promiscuity but I had been talking about saving lives by advocating safe sex practices. I was very angry that they should try and put a guilt trip on me with their emotional blackmail. Their attitude didn't make sense despite my attempts at rational discussion so we had very little contact with each other over the next couple of years and I continued to do whatever press interviews I felt were necessary to promote my business but I never told my parents about them.

There is an interesting postscript to this story in that just recently I appeared on a lifestyle television program talking about the new erotica for women and mentioned it to my mother in an attempt to see if her views had softened over the years. To my surprise she referred back to the previous episode by remarking that she couldn't cope with me talking about violence! I tried to explain that I had been talking about safe sex. It emerged that she obviously hadn't heard a word I'd said on the interview because she'd shut off at the mere mention of the term X rated videos which she equates to violence. I find this very disturbing because in Australia X rated videos contain absolutely no violence whatsoever and only portray consensual sexual activity. I am astonished that someone like my mother, who has a vested interest (me) in being informed of the censorship laws, should be so ignorant.

I know I will never be able to convince my parents that what I do is "okay" so I have to come to terms with the fact that I can't discuss my business with them as it causes them such distress. This is unfortunate as I'm sure I'm not alone in hoping for the approval of my parents.

I enjoy my work very much and we are now launching a new catalogue of erotic products for women and couples featuring videos, books, lingerie, aromatherapy products, vibrators and other miscellaneous sex toys. The adult industry is a very exciting and challenging area to be working in and one of the best things about it is that we are providing a much needed service for people and I find I learn something new every day . . . long may it continue!

Helen Ryles is a blind and deaf woman living in England. She is active in many different projects, including writing. Unfortunately, her piece is very short. This is probably due to the lack of pornography available for people with such disabilities.

Pornography

Helen Ryles

I have had very little contact with pornography. Once, when I was sighted, I saw some pictures of naked women with their legs wide open on a public footpath. I felt this was really disgusting. I picked it up and hid it out of public vision. Since then I've not really had much to do with pornography of that nature. I certainly don't miss it; neither am I against it.

The connection that the religious groups and certain feminists make between pornography and violence is false. There isn't really a connection between provocative clothes and rape. A woman who was dressed like a Muslim woman, alone in a dark deserted place, would be at just as much risk as a woman in sexy clothing. Like most criminals, rapists will try to choose safe targets. This is why children and old people are sometimes at risk.

I have a friend who says he reads pornography sometimes. I've been with him for a year now. He has many opportunities to make me have sex with him. He hasn't tried. On the other hand, I was raped once by a man from Saudi Arabia. Pornography is banned there.

What would concern me most if pornography was banned is that a lot of people cannot distinguish between sex education and pornography. Countries that ban pornography usually ban sex education as well. I once wrote a letter to a braille magazine about sex outside marriage. It said:

As regards to Frank Routzen's letter (he wrote to say that nobody should be having sex before marriage), I feel that it's all very well for some. As a multi-disabled person I feel the chances of me getting married to an interesting and caring person is very, very slim. I don't believe in fairy tales.

I have also been told sex outside marriage was bad, and casual lovers are even worse. However, I disagree. While I know cases of people getting divorced after only three months, I also know a case of a couple living ten years together without being married. Marriage will not make people stick together; far from it. In some cases, the responsibility and return to reality is what can cause a split and later a divorce. If one is to get married, one should have shared interests, the same sort of background, and total compatibility and commitment with one's partner.

This relationship does not offer itself to everyone. Some people are committed to a job or because of character defects, or because of a mental or physical disability. Does this mean people in this group have to be deprived of one of the best experiences in life (sex)? To some people, the idea of sex between two people who are not and have no intention of getting married is very shocking. Even more so if one of the persons happens to be disabled. The normal person gets accused of using the disabled person, as if the disabled person did not know what was going on.

However, I agree that partners/lovers should not tell lies. It is lies that hurt when a relationship breaks down, not sex.

I had a lot of response to this letter. Many accused me of sleeping out with all and sundry. They said I would end up with AIDS as God's punishment. A reader even described it as rank pornography. Fortunately, I did get a couple of positive responses in the magazine, as well as from a lot of my pen pals who read this magazine.

RNIB have a braille magazine called *Alpha*, for women, which has erotic articles in it. Many of the blind write in to say how good these articles are — that they only wish that it was around when they were younger. I, too, have found it useful. I learnt that I wasn't the only woman in the world to masturbate, and that it was so common that there was even such a thing as sex toys. *Alpha* also has letters complaining about the pornography in it.

I feel that sex education and having a guilt-free attitude towards sex are vitally important. Sex education should start very early. It should also include lessons in self-defense. What to do if a strange man/boy approaches (where to strike if he's making unwelcome approaches), how and why to refuse a boyfriend who won't wear a condom, or just basically knowing one has a right to say "No", even if the request for sex is accompanied by lots of expensive presents. One should also learn that one has a right to say yes and not feel guilty about it. I feel that the bad experiences I've had of sex could have been avoided (even the rape) if I'd known more about sex and about self-defense.

Rowan Green is twenty seven and lives in London with two cats and a fast-breeding second hand book collection. Current ambitions are to have some of her fiction published and to improve her needlework.

The Phantom in the Closet

Rowan Green

Everything changed for me at seven years of age. That's when my family moved to a new town. Somehow I failed to make new friends. I spent the rest of my school career being bullied, or alone. As such I missed out on the usual playground gossip. I spent years putting my toilet paper in sanitary disposal bins. When the girls got taken for a sex education class at eleven, it was a total revelation. My mother had told me that babies occurred "When people love each other". Having been raised in a science-fiction mad household I assumed she meant some form of telepathy.

Sex was not treated in a negative way in my family, it was just not talked about. Sex was in the closet — literally. Sometime in my early teens I discovered that behind the clothes in my parents' bedroom closet there was a pile of magazines; mostly *Forum*, but a few *Penthouse* and *Mayfair*. I spent many hours reading them during the next years. I had my first orgasm after reading how, and knew what fellatio was long before I could pronounce it. I became a sexual expert, in theory at least.

At the real thing, I was a slow starter. I put my early crushes on other girls down to a "homosexual phase" (as I said, I was a bit of an expert). Later, I developed a reassuring interest in Steven Spielberg, though I now realize it was mental rather than physical. Falling in love with a female friend when I was 17 came as a complete surprise. I didn't think it was bad, but it shook up my self image. Until then I'd not been interested in actually having sex, but now I wanted to explore my sexuality. I determined to lose my virginity before I was 18. In fact it happened a couple of weeks after my birthday. I slept with a very sweet guy — older, but also a virgin — an experience which was physically pleasant but emotionally uninvolving. A few months later I had my first experience with a woman, in a bender at Greenham Common. It was physically a little disappointing (well it was very vanilla ... *), but I fell madly in love. She wasn't interested in a relationship though.

Nine years on I've been through several relationships, a polytechnic course, homelessness, and a period of celibacy. So, has reading porn in my teenage years turned me into a sex-mad pervert? I don't think I've been sex-mad — I've had a fair few sexual disasters, but not compulsive sexual activity. As for being a pervert — well, I am one (as long as it's safe and consensual I'll consider doing it), but I think that has more to do with nine years of isolation and torture as a child — which is what I consider my experience of bullying to have been. I'm into power and trust games as a way of confronting the emotional damage of my past, not because my passions have been unnaturally inflamed. I'd have to distinguish between the magazines I read as well. The mainstream, softcore mags I really remember very little about. They were occasionally a turn-on, but mostly plain boring. *Forum* was more interesting, and provided me with knowledge that allowed me to approach actually doing sex with basic good sense and without fear. It has contributed to the open attitude to sex which has helped me to accept my sexual self.

When I hear the arguments against porn, a lot of them seem convincing. Yet they don't fit with my own experience. I've seen dull, repetitive, mass-market rubbish, and intelligent, informative alternatives. That the alternatives can't get wider distribution seems much more of a problem than the innocuous tripe being peddled on most top shelves. You hear of women being exploited

---

* Editor's note: Not sadomasochistic.

and even raped, but don't office bosses rape their secretaries too? A world in which women could report such abuses, and get support from the legal system, would do more to help than forcing the industry underground. The sex workers I've known (quite large numbers) seem to want better working conditions, not state attacks on the industry and their livelihoods. We need to empower sex workers, not attempt to save them from themselves and take away their freedom of choice in the process.

If we are worried about the effect on vulnerable minds, we need to teach them to distinguish between fantasy and reality. Images of rape and violence are surely not crimes equivalent to real rape and violence, yet current restrictions on the distribution of images seem to treat them as such. Blurring this distinction seems dangerous to me. We also need to be able to talk openly about sex, in order to pass on information to keep ourselves safe and healthy. HIV is an obvious issue, but this also applies to S/M practices. I recently saw photographs of the making of a porn film, which showed a woman (appearing quite happy) with her hands raised in handcuffs and whip marks scattered across her back. You might like to argue that in an ideal world nobody would want S/M, but in the meanwhile I wish someone had told the participants that hard edges on handcuffs can cause nerve damage, and you shouldn't whip someone on the kidney area and spine . . . Though with major shop chains refusing to stock any magazine which deals with S/M, who is going to tell them? Seeing images like this makes me want to see more openness, not less.

I'm now entering a new phase in my relationship with porn- becoming a producer as well as a consumer. After my years of homelessness, I've now got a secure base, and am beginning to express myself through writing. I'm finding that erotic stories, though not all I write, are a major part of my output. Perhaps because I spent much of my childhood without positive communications with other humans, it's very important to me to express my feelings — to be heard, and not to shut up because someone else doesn't like the truth about my, and perhaps their, feelings.

I've been told so many times that I'm fat, ugly, smelly, pathetic, etc. that it became difficult to tell the truth from the insults and lies. Writing out my fantasies is a way of facing my fears and cutting through those lies and insults. Showing my stories to other people is a way of throwing off the false shame which has been imposed on me by my tormentors.

Showing a story to someone else for the first time is a terrifying moment. It means exposing myself and trusting that it won't be used as an opportunity to attack me, as I have been attacked many times in my life. A positive reaction is a relief and an affirmation. In this context, censorship, which was just an occasional irritant before, has become a personal threat. I write to be honest, to be true to myself and hopefully to give pleasure to others. While my stories fall within current legal bounds, the thought that a rumour that I was producing something 'unacceptable' might lead to my home being raided, possessions seized, family shamed etc., is frankly scary. I'm not being exploited, nor am I exploiting anyone else, so what is the problem?

It seems that much of the common reaction to porn comes down to fear. People don't want to confront the 'nasty' things in life, or even hear about them; a case of ignoring both reality and messenger, and shooting the message. They're afraid of contamination, yet so much of what they are avoiding is not what they believe it to be. A few days ago, I showed a fellow student, a respectable woman, copies of some of the magazines the big chains won't stock. She was very reluctant to look, but when finally persuaded she seemed perhaps a little let down. She even described the Lesbian magazine *Quim* as "A bit *Girl's Own*" (not a description I'd use!).

People are wasting energy creating ghosts to be afraid of. It is only when we accept our fantasies as harmless phantoms that we can direct this mental energy to dealing with reality.

Linzi Drew began her 'showbiz' career in 1976 as a cheerleader for Bristol City Football Club. After some national press coverage, she was spotted by the tabloid newspapers, and shortly after embarked upon a career as a glamour model, appearing on 'page 3' and numerous calendars. Drew's popularity with the punters prompted the editor of girlie magazine Club International *to offer her a regular monthly column, and in 1987 she was headhunted by* Penthouse *magazine (UK) and enrolled as their first female editor. Her own series of sexy videos has been well-received; the first, 'I Love Linzi,' sold 45,000 in just three months. In 1992, she was given a four-month prison sentence for possession of obscene material for gain. Her most recent book is an autobiography,* Try Everything Once, Except Incest and Morris Dancing.

Adventures in Pornoland

Linzi Drew

My first face to face experience of erotica was a copy of a *Fiesta* magazine that I found at home when I was about sixteen or seventeen years old. My Father wasn't in the habit of buying girlie magazines, but he was a private landlord and occasionally when a tenant moved out such things were left behind, and somehow or other ended up at home.

I recall discovering this 'naughty' magazine amongst a pile of old papers in the sun lounge. It immediately caught my interest, but as I flicked through, I wasn't in the least bit taken with the photographs of scantily clad models, although they didn't shock or repulse me. What thrilled and fascinated me were the sexy stories, mainly the readers' letters. Those intimate, carnal confessions of rampant sex in the woods, or torrid tales of blow jobs in the next door neighbour's Ford Anglia, made me feel hot and set my pussy throbbing.

I'd wait until my parents went out, seek out the well-thumbed copy of Fiesta and lie on the floor in our sun lounge. As I read it from cover to cover, my groin would start to throb. I'd usually bring myself off by grinding my pussy against the hard, carpeted floor.

Since that first wet, joyous experience, almost two decades ago, I have perused hundreds, if not thousands of similar girlie magazines. These days I have my own letters magazine, *Linzi Drew's EROS*, which is packed full of naked girlies and page after page of explicit letters. I look at the sensual, alluring models spread eagled over each glossy page, and although I have very strong bisexual tendencies, I tend to view these lovelies with no more than professional eye. Static images on a printed page have never really done that much for my libido. The salacious stories and lewd letters, on the other hand, still make me wet between the legs! When hard at work selecting readers' letters for inclusion in *EROS* magazine. I find some of them so arousing that I have to stop working at my PC, lie down on the floor of my office and have a good wank. Alternatively, if my boyfriend's around, I demand he stop what he's doing immediately and come and lick my pussy that instant! Often we end up fucking right there and then on the floor, which always makes for a pleasant interlude during my working day.

Magazines are fun, but my favourite form of porn is on video. I find moving images of sex play much more stimulating. I love watching lesbian videos as I'm very into girls at the moment, which is hardly surprising as I always seem to be in the company of beautiful young models wearing next to nothing.

On video I love to watch two women kissing, their tongues wild as they swirl in and out of each other's hot, eager mouths. I like the action to be slow and languid as one lover begins to strip the other, cups her breasts, kisses her swollen pink nipples and moves agonizingly slowly down over her belly. I love to see a woman slowly and seductively strip her female partner, slide a hand inside damp panties, and at this point I find it more exciting if for a moment or two I can't actually see what's going on, just imagine. When her knickers are eventually pulled off to the side, or peeled down her legs, I long to see firm hands, complete with manicured, long, painted fingernails, grip splayed thighs. Watching beautiful hands spread wet pussy lips is always a great turn on for me, and of course when fingers and a tongue slide between those pink pulsating lovelips I like to see all the action.

Lesbian videos that see women being shafted by bloody great dildos do little for me, I far prefer stimulation to be soft and gentle. Most of the lesbian vids that turn me on would be classed as hardcore and therefore not legal in this country. But I do find some of the softcore lesbian videos a turn on. For instance I shot quite a lot of girl/girl scenes for my 'Members Only' video series and when choosing girls to work together, I always tried to seek out models who weren't just performing girl/girl sex for the cash, and because they thought it an easy option, but rather because they fancied licking pussy! That way, although the BBFC prohibit any explicit pussy shots, the girls can still really get off on each other, and their real, orgasmic enjoyment affords us, the video viewer, the knowledge that even if the erotic image is framed so you can't quite see that probing tongue snaking between trembling lovelips, you know damn well it's going in there!

Recently I made a softcore film for this country called 'I Love Linzi Too'. In the second sequence I have a scene with this unbelievably beautiful French teenager. She's called Draghixa, is nineteen, has dark blonde, corkscrewed hair, a fabulous body, long fingernails and the most amazing tits I've ever had the pleasure to clamp my mouth around. I'm getting carried away here! She also has just won best European actress at the 1995 Cannes Porn Awards. Anyway prior to my lesbian lickings with the lovely Draghixa, I begin the video by lying on a sun lounger in the glorious Spanish sunshine playing with myself. Not a bad way to make a living, you might think, and I have to agree! Unbeknown to me, my masturbatory performance was having one hell of an effect on the mouthwatering Draghixa. Once I'd brought myself to climax, my make-up artist came to powder my nose and good-naturedly whispered to me that my antics were driving Draghixa crazy. She told me the lovely Frenchie just wouldn't sit still to have her make-up done, because she was far too interested in watching me having a wank, so consequently kept running out onto the balcony to get a better look! That did my ego the power of good, not to mention had me panting to get at her!

Our scene together was so fucking sexy. When we finished filming, my boyfriend, the cameraman, and her boyfriend, a porn stud, went off for a beer together and left me and Draghixa to continue our cunt-kissing in peace! So although the lesbian sex scene was shot for a softcore video, it was for real. So to say I only find hardcore lesbian videos a turn on isn't strictly true. I do find some softcore videos arousing, just as long as I know the action is for real, not simulated. That way I don't feel cheated.

But my personal preferences on porn aside, I cannot for the life of me understand this country's outdated pornography laws. Why we have to talk of softcore and hardcore, when I believe the majority of the adult population in this country don't really know what we 'pornsters' are on about! They just want to watch real sex and be titillated! Softcore pornography is generally tits and bums, limp penises and fucking when you can't actually see penetration. Every magazine still has to be carefully scrutinized by distributors and lawyers, and every video frame examined by the British Board of Film Classification. I admit that the new breed of women's magazines that feature gorgeous hunks stark naked are a great step forward, but what pisses me off immensely is the fact that we are only permitted to ogle these handsome creatures in the raw providing they haven't got a stiffy! I can only assume that the 'powers that be' believe that allowing us to view an erect penis would prove dangerous! It's laughable isn't it? And with video productions, the rules are no less nonsensical. I remember actually having to cut a scene from one boy/girl video that I produced because I was told that it looked like they were enjoying it too much! Surely you can't enjoy sex too much!

But it's no laughing matter when you actually get sent to prison because of our archaic, outdated porn laws. My boyfriend, Lindsay Honey, ran a small mail order porn company which serviced less than one hundred punters. Unfortunately while he was away in America I collected his mail on one occasion. The following morning at the crack of dawn my house was taken apart by five officers of the obscene publications squad, whose eyes lit up when they spotted me! For such a minor role in such a heinous crime, I received a four month prison sentence which was bad enough, but my boyfriend was treated even more outrageously; he was given nine months in jail. And for what? For supplying consenting adults with videos that depicted images of other consenting adults screwing. If a nice police officer from the OPS hadn't spent four years buying some of these hardcore videos, of a type freely available in every other member state of the EC, a great deal of taxpayers' money wouldn't have been chucked down the drain, and I wouldn't have ended up in Holloway nick*!

Being sent to prison for assisting my other half in running a porno company is probably my only bad experience of pornography, which I suppose is pretty good when you consider that I've been in the business of selling sex in one way or another for around a decade and a half. Although I spend most of my working life surrounded by porno images and raunchy readers' writes, I enjoy my work and enjoy my sex life. And as both my partner and I work closely together in this field, I certainly don't have any problems with him looking at pornography. On the contrary, he spends half his life looking at other females 'naughty bits' through a camera lens, and that's fine by me! I do wish more men and women in this country would stand up and unashamedly

---

* UK slang for prison.

admit that they get turned on by a bit of porn, but I do understand that it can be extremely difficult because of the sexually repressed society we live in. I believe we should be able to talk candidly about the pleasure pornography can bring, without fear of reproach. If we could, then perhaps our outdated obscenity laws might be relaxed? Because to my mind, more erotica available on the open market makes for a better choice for all us consenting adults who love a bit of porn!

Jen Durbin is the pen name for a teacher/writer/administrator who lives and works in the San Francisco Bay Area. Durbin earned her Ph.D. from the University of California at Berkeley in 1990. This spring she is teaching her Women's Studies class on "Feminism and Pornography" for the fourth time. Durbin is a frequent contributor of feature articles and book reviews to the San Francisco Bay Area's weekly sex magazine, Spectator, *in which this essay first appeared. She lives with her beautiful, talented lover and her beautiful, down-to-earth twenty-one-year-old daughter. This female household revolves around a small acrobatic dog named Buster, who is so famous on campus that he will blow Durbin's cover if any of the readers of this collection are students or faculty there.*

Confessions of a Feminist Porn Teacher

Jen Durbin

A riddle: who watches a lot of porn, talks a lot about porn, and even writes a lot of porn, but has never masturbated to a fuck film? Well, one answer might be Andrea Dworkin. Another would be me. I teach a course called "Feminism and Pornography" at a local university. When I first created this course two years ago, I had no idea what I was getting myself into. I had thought I would be teaching in the English Department, but I was informed at the last minute that I needed to design a Women's Studies course, so I massaged the syllabus on banned books that I had prepared, creating a course on pornography. I had been writing pornography for private audiences (mainly anyone I was trying to seduce) for about a dozen years, but I had had limited experience with video porn and even less experience with the considerable controversy surrounding porn.

I had a lot to learn, and fast. Our class became an exploring party, an expedition into the world of sexually explicit material.

My students and I read the arguments of feminists who are against pornography, feminists who are against censorship, and feminists who are in favour of pornography. More importantly, we read and viewed pornography for ourselves. It's too easy to get a skewed impression of porn if you only read about it. Students who read Andrea Dworkin become convinced that pornography equals pictures of dead Asian women hanging from trees, smiling buxom women meeting a gruesome fate in a meat grinder, ecstatic women fellating revolvers, etc. Students who read Nina Hartley become convinced that pornography is a form of self-actualization for uninhibited feminists. If they have no direct experience on which to base an independent opinion, the students' opinions will be largely determined by the relative persuasive powers of Dworkin or Hartley, both of whom, by the way, derive the force of their very different arguments in part from the abnormally large volume of porn they themselves have screened.

So we watch and read a lot of porn together. This simple statement surprises a lot of people. Some find it inappropriate for a university course. They forget that no professor would expect freshmen to write essays on art history or the reproductive organs of amphibians without ever having seen a painting or a frog. I assign several formal essays in the course of the semester, and I feel obliged to provide something for my budding scholars to analyse first hand.

Some people squirm at the idea of watching sexually explicit videos in groups. This surprises me, because they are very likely the same people who have watched porn in groups themselves, at bachelor's parties, fraternities, and the like. "What," they ask, "do you do if someone gets, ah, aroused? Isn't it embarrassing?" I reply that so far that has not come up, so to speak. Our viewing sessions feel very different from the viewing sessions at the Pink Pussycat. We usually spend a lot of time fighting over the remote control: one faction inevitably wants to fast forward through the fucking and sucking to get to some dialogue, and once we hear the quality of the dialogue, another very vocal group will want to fast forward through the dialogue to get to the fucking and sucking. But no matter whether we are watching plunging organs or listening to bad dialogue, we are operating in an analytical mode. My students' voices fill the room, as they comment on stereotypes, anomalies, and implied messages. And we laugh a lot. If you've never noticed that porn is pretty comical, you must not be paying attention.

Arousal is actually one of the least likely responses during our viewing sessions. It's just too damned crowded. Everyone is naturally very aware of each other's and their own need for personal space in such a crowd, and no one (as far as I can tell) checks anyone else's faces or crotches for signs of arousal, expecting the same modicum of privacy in return. I guess it's the same etiquette that dictates where men direct their gazes in a urinal.

Of course, no one's response to porn is purely analytical— and if ours were, we would be missing the point.

So if you confess to sneaking an occasional tiny peek, just out of curiosity, at your neighbour in the urinal, I will admit I occasionally get aroused when watching video porn in a group setting. And I'm sure that if pressed, each of my students would confess to the same thing. And although we learn a lot from watching porn and analysing it, I believe we learn even more from looking at our own interactions with the world of porn.

Considering that well over one hundred X-rated films are produced each year in Los Angeles alone, it's probably safe to say that very few people are qualified to make accurate generalizations about the entire genre. So when I hear, for example, that porn is becoming progressively more violent, I must first ask who identified this trend . . . and what might have motivated that person to choose the films he or she considered representative of the genre. Early in the spring semester, my class was reading the work of the anti-porn feminists. I wanted to give them an idea of the kind of pornography these writers objected to, so I asked each group to rent the most offensive movie they could find. Most of the students responded to this assignment with variations on a single theme: same-sex sado-masochism. The difference between the students' idea of offensive and Dworkin/MacKinnon's idea was instructive. What we learned about Dworkin and MacKinnon was pretty trivial; what was less trivial was confronting our own homophobia.

I have seen lots of students grow and change during the course of the semester. And to tell you the truth, I don't care in which direction they grow, as long as they are keeping an open mind. You often hear people celebrated for having the courage of their convictions. I too celebrate that quality in my students, while also realizing that sometimes it takes even more courage to change one's convictions. I had one student who started out the semester with the idea that all pornography was harmful and degrading to women. Rebecca even stood up at a meeting called "Everything You Ever Wanted to Know About Sex Workers", and confronted Miki Demarest with an issue of *The Spectator*, which Miki edited in those days. "'Cum on me, shoot your load all over my face, stick it up my ass,'" read Rebecca. "This view of women as sex objects is the very thing that I, as a feminist have been working against all my life. How can you, who call yourself a feminist, contribute to this treatment of women?" It was an honest cry from the heart, one that required a lot of courage, considering the sur-roundings: nearly one hundred women in the sex industry who were almost militantly proud of their careers.

I was proud of Rebecca that night for having the courage of her convictions in a place where her opinion would not be popular, and as the semester progressed I realized that she had the second kind of courage as well. As soon as she began think-ing hard about the subject, she inevitably realized that no simple formula or slogan could accurately account for pornography. In a quest for something closer to the truth about porn, Rebecca took on a special research project: she interviewed several sex work-ers and really listened to what they had to say. One of the women she spoke to was a dominatrix. This led Rebecca to attend an S/M lecture/demonstration. Her research expanded past the words and lives of others to include a look inside herself.

Within a couple of months, her classroom persona shifted radically. During a discussion of pornography versus erotica, she called me on my biases: "I know," she said, "Erotica is anything you like and pornography is anything I like." Each of us learned a lesson from her apparent wisecrack: from that day forward I dropped the elitist euphemism for the sexually explicit material I read and write, and she acknowledged that she had more in common with the sex workers than she had initially realized. In her final essay for the semester she argued that although it was sometimes hard to distinguish between women's expressions of their own sexuality and women parroting male versions of female sexuality, we will never be able to make that distinction as long as we are unwilling to listen to women — all kinds of women — speaking about sex in the first place.

Another student, whom I'll call Tammy, enrolled in my class because she was eager to argue with the feminists. She had an idea that a Women's Studies course on feminism and pornography would attract a bunch of humourless prudes who looked upon women as helpless victims of the patriarchy. I don't really blame her for her expectations, which had been carefully molded by a mass media that prefers cartoon feminist villains to anyone whose ideas are too complex to make a big, immediate, cartoon BANG! Even the reporters who are sympathetic to feminism too often want to present the same cartoon figures, but dressed up as comic-book heroines instead. When the new adult night-club, Centerfolds, opened recently in San Francisco, a well-intentioned reporter from KGO called and invited me to appear on a broadcast from the nightclub. She said that Centerfolds' owners would be there praising adult entertainment, and they needed someone who would point out how degrading it was for the women. She assumed that because I was a feminist, that would be my stance. I told her I hadn't seen the place yet, so I couldn't possibly have formed an opinion. I also told her that an anti-porn feminist is a rare species in the Bay Area, and recommended that she take the Centerfolds broadcast as an opportunity to present a more balanced view of the feminist response to pornography.

A more balanced spectrum was what Tammy actually found when she came into my class, spoiling for a fight with the feminists. If her fellow students, most of whom identify themselves as feminists, had been prudes, they never would have signed up for the class. If they had been humourless, they never would have survived it. Camille Paglia gets a lot of attention for blaming feminists for turning women into helpless victims, but her incoherent rhetoric would not carry her far in the rigorous class discussions among my students, who are learning to think for themselves, which is the best protection against victimization. At the end of the semester we had a class party. One of the students suggested that each person announce why he or she had taken the class in the first place. Tammy said, "I came here to kick some feminist butt. But to my surprise I learned that I am a feminist." She's right. She has the passion and humour and commitment that characterize the feminists whom watchers of mass media unfortunately never see.

A lot of my students end up thinking that everyone should take a course like mine, and who am I to disagree? Of course I believe in the importance of education, and of the free speech that is nurtured in the university classroom. But to tell the truth, you probably don't need a class on porn to help you examine your culture and yourself. The average reader of *Spectator*[11] has watched enough stroke films to support a quite sophisticated analysis not only of porn and mass media, but also of his or her own psyche. Of course not everyone wants to start analysing what turns them on and why. They may fear that if they open

---

[11] Author's note: This essay first appeared in the *Spectator*, the San Francisco Bay Area's weekly sex news magazine.

up their libidos and start peering and poking around in there, they might damage the delicate mechanism.

Well, I'll tell you what I tell people who ask how teaching a porn class has affected my sex life. After the first few weeks, I was so overwhelmed by graphic close-ups of pimply, pulsating organs that I felt nauseated at the mere thought of having sex. In addition to the gut reaction, I was experiencing the fate of the centipede who could not walk any more once he stopped to think about which leg followed which. As anyone can tell you, over analysis can be a pretty potent antidote to spontaneous passion. One of my students lamented that she could no longer have sex without being conscious of the political implications of the positions of her and her lover's bodies. The difference between humans and other animals became impossible to ignore: we cannot check our cultural baggage at the door before climbing into bed, or into a sling hanging from the ceiling, for that matter.

Of course, this is only a disadvantage if fucking like animals is the highest goal. Humans have certain advantages when it comes to sex. For instance, we don't have to wait for mating season. And it turns out that the human brain is not a sexual liability but an asset — in fact, it's a nearly infinite erogenous zone. And an examination of that zone is just as likely to result in the discovery of whole new territories as it is to render some old familiar territories defunct. If a person discovers, for instance, that the feel of chains on her wrists reminds her of her political oppression, that discovery might enhance the pleasure she takes in testing or challenging the limits of her bondage in a playful, safe environment. Or she may find that the chains have lost their power to arouse her, freeing her to find a new source of arousal, perhaps in her own strength. Either way, in the final analysis she will have learned something valuable and enhanced her sex life.

It's a truism that one of the uses of pornography is to give people new ideas of what to do in bed. But anyone who watches much x-rated material can tell you that it's pretty formulaic — it can give one the stifling sensation that there is nothing new under the sun. I suspect that many viewers find that most scenes leave them cold, while some scenes make them uncomfortable and other scenes generate guaranteed fireworks. Certainly that's why remote controls were invented. But I've been learning that my discomfort can be just as worthwhile, though perhaps not as immediately satisfying, as the fireworks. Sometimes just identifying the source of my discomfort gives me something as simple yet essential as the ability to say no. And sometimes my discomfort suggests a course of political action. At other times I realize that my own comfort zone is too tight for me, so I let out the seams to make room for all the growth I have experienced teaching pornography to a bunch of freshmen and sophomores.

Along with another active FAC member, Cherie Matrix (stage named Cherry Cakemix) formed Dragon Ladies in the spring of 1995. They have organised and produced their own vaudevillian revues exploring the issues of sexual politics by examining female rudeness on stage. Matrix also works for Obsolete, a London based company that builds web sites for the Internet and curates Backspace, their virtual gallery.

Matrix has modeled for well known photographers, appearing in many body art and manipulation publications. She does subscribe to the western beauty myth that 'blondes have more fun', but also believes there are more beautiful, pagan and primitive ways to enhance the body.

Access: All Areas

Cherie Matrix

I was always quite blasé about pornography. It has always been accessible to me and I took it for granted that it would be available wherever my family lived, although sometimes it did take a bit of searching. My taste is incredibly varied, yet I am also very choosy when it comes to what I consider arousing material. I am a voracious consumer of products I get pleasure from. Because of this, I used to feel that anti-censorship as a wider campaign topic was more important than focusing on pornography.

Then, at a Humanist meeting, I heard the Feminists Against Censorship argument and realized another part of my life, just like my right to silence, was under threat by government legislation. I became involved in FAC and the fight against the anti-porn campaigners soon after that Humanist meeting. My main reason for becoming involved is that I have always enjoyed pornography, and do not want to be classed as a criminal because of this harmless enjoyment.

There are numerous more important topics that should be addressed by government. Censorship is an obvious waste of the judiciary's time, as well as the state's funds. Taxes pay for the censorship of what is "pornographic". Safe sex guides, art, music, and classic literature are all attacked by the contemporary "moral" campaigners.

Out of all the varied sexual images that I enjoy, my main interests throughout my life have been sexy vampires, muscular women and the depiction of pain. In recent years, my favourite sex-pages have been in magazines with sexually powerful depictions of muscular women with guns, vampires and informative features on role playing. I have used many of the photographs as a springboard for my fantasies. My not so exceptional gun-fuck fantasy has been enhanced enormously by the sight of a topless woman with two uzi-type guns crossed over her bare breasts.

It was inevitable that I would discover the pages of *Fangoria* when I was younger because it is a magazine dedicated to all those grisly special effects in horror movies that got me tingly with excitement. I bought it (along with National Geographic) for fashion tips, like how to look good while tying people up, etc. At college, I watched every horror movie I could and studied their arousing effects along with my Human Sexuality course. The cycle of life=sex as the easiest way to deny death, wrapped up in cosmetic special effects is the most sexually dynamic imagery available on screen.

My sexual obsession with portrayals of gore actually came in handy once I had moved to London from the US and hooked up with a beautifully tattooed bisexual skinhead named Stephanie. She claimed to have gotten an alleged snuff video. This video, quite unbelievably, had supposedly been found in an alley by a street sweeper! (Yes, it was rubbish.)

I had no feelings of anticipation leading up to viewing the "snuff" film, mostly because I doubted its genuineness and at that point in my life I had never seen a proper pornographic film that excited me. The idea of sitting through another "violent" porn video with women as victims both bored and enraged me, as well. As soon as the video started I could tell all the blood was fake. The actors had learned all their facial expressions from Hammer House of Horror. I had viewed more believable (and sexy) supposed death scenes and torture on late night television, using more elaborate special effects. This video had no effect whatsoever.

The British Government has become increasingly strict on the rental and sale of "video nastys". I have always felt it should be the opposite. The more people realize the extent of what is achieved with special effects on video and film, the less likely they are to believe in the urban myths of snuff films produced in the US and UK.

Many years before the "snuff" film incident, while at some fashionable punk/art-fuck party in a impressive beachside apartment, I came across the photograph that made me a devoted fan of muscular, sexy horror. It was published in a mainstream US men's porn magazine, probably *Hustler*. The photo was of two topless and muscular, obviously lesbian, vampires locked in a relentless embrace. I had to have this page. No longer do I remember if I asked for permission to possess it. I ripped that page from the magazine and carried the photograph around the world with me for years, until I became worried about its condition and hung it on my wall. For many years, I used the imagery of the lesbian vampires to 'bate[12] and still fantasize about it. I can still get wet thinking about all the previous pleasure that photo has given me. The taste and texture of a woman's quivering neck has never looked so appetizing.

All due to this one page, ripped from a porn mag, blood became my sexuality and vamp became my fashion statement. I was the sexiest tattooed skinhead in a corset that ever shopped LA's infamous sex emporium, The Pleasure Chest. On one shop-

---

[12] Short for "masturbate". Handy slang you can use at home.

ping expedition, accompanied by my favourite pierced surfer, I wandered the aisles of LA's best sex shop fingering the dildos and being as blasé' about the whole atmosphere as usual. Another 'bate photo — an arty black and white muscular nude sitting on a hard floor, yet loosely wrapped in barbed wire. I did not need to possess this photo, the memory was enough.

The person in the photo looked very tranquil, without a glimpse of pain. I never discovered if the barbed wire was real. However, the imagery of that photograph enhanced my fascination with and arousal at the idea of depictions of discomfort. I have imagined the barbed wire digging into tattooed skin at exact intervals; covering arms, legs, body, and even face and lips, although this part was free of wire in the photograph.

I have gotten a lot of fantasy mileage out of photos and they've allowed me the chance to come safely to terms with my sexuality. S/M role playing had been inherent since I was very young. Even though I hadn't suppressed my sadistic urges, the barbed wire was the first imagery that reinforced that these feelings could be beautiful. My sex scenes were now elevated to art.

For awhile, still influenced by the black+white still, barbed wire became my craft. I tattooed it on skin, and used it in shows. Gloriously, a pornographic image influenced many aspects of my varied life.

I have always found women's bodies more attractive than men's bodies. However, even though pornography was very accessible, the women on the pages of most pornographic magazines were not the type I found attractive. I wanted to see athletic women with muscular bodies like in my cherished vamp photo. Women whose physiques encased *real* power — not just sexual attraction, but real strength. Even the ex-cheerleaders in Playboy-type publications seemed to have slimmed so radically that they had lost the definition of those cheerleader leg muscles, but gained silicon pom-poms!

I waded through page after page of sports magazines, particularly surfing, to gaze longingly at all that upper body strength glistening in the sun. Probably around the same time, I found the first image of a man that stimulated me enough to want to have sex with one. It was a surfing spread in my mother's *Playgirl*. Luckily, we lived in the US, so we actually got to see an erection. I remember that *Playgirl* quite vividly. We had a pile at the house, so it's not remembered for its rarity. It is not anything I have fantasized about during sex, even though the memory gets me tingling in all the right, pierced, places.

The surfing photos are examples that I have seen and taken notice of many types of sexuality. A great deal of my life has been spent in the company of surfers and I have been attracted to a few and madly, passionately in love with my favourite. I cannot tell if that was due to the imagery I found arousing or just spending most of my life in Southern California.

If I lived in a different part of the world where censorship against pornography is even stricter, I may never have discovered what I feel to be such positive sexual imagery. I am sure I would have found other images to 'bate over. However, even though I realize I was directly influenced, I may not have ever felt either sexually or intellectually fulfilled.

In the '90s, due to lowered video and printing costs, stylized porn has become more accessible as prices have come down. Over the last few years, I have viewed many videos of athletic and beautiful women performing sex acts in architecturally pleasant surroundings, some even by the beach! The stereotypical woman as victim image is being pushed aside increasingly. In its place I am happy to see women of all sizes and colours being assertive. This type of video pornography has been available since the advent of video. It is only now that the type of porn I like to view has become affordable to me.

While pornography is stylized to more diverse tastes, other media forms seem to be using more softcore sexual imagery in there products. Both men's and women's fashion magazines, as well as current affairs periodicals, are all using more than the basic cheesecake in their features. And don't even talk to me about porn on the Internet! The few poor quality images I've managed to find are so mainstream and boring that I've given up trying to download any porn off the web. But it's just a matter of time before I can fashion my own!!

So, even though beautiful pornography is more widely available, it is the chance encounters with thimble-sized nipples on a sandy beach, see-through trashy underclothes on a butch, tattooed model, and other such provocative images in well-known highly distributed fashion glossies that my mind keeps wandering back to.

Marcelle Perks is a student on an MA Media Studies course in London, England, where she is currently researching British horror cinema. Perks is one of very few female journalists writing about horror films. She has previously worked for a video production company, an arts cinema and an advertising agency.

DIY Pornography

Marcelle Perks

I have no professional involvement with the sex industry except as an occasional writer for various top shelf publications such as *Redeemer* and *Videoworld*. However, as a woman, even my very presence in such texts (regardless of actual content) puts question marks on my integrity for those who find pornography immoral or anti-feminist. It seems every time I tell someone what I do, I have to defend the right to consume and participate in what is perceived as a men-only club.

I've been running up against this kind of attitude ever since my breasts made an early appearance when I was twelve years old. The coming of my curves became a sign that I was 'easy' just as at fifteen my bleach blonde hair meant I couldn't possibly be a virgin. The male population seems to prefer women to look like sex objects but not to feel sexy. When some feminist groups try to censor pornography, it is reaction, not resistance. Pornography unquestionably endorses many negative stereotypes but the right to consume and create our own pornography is essential if we are to emerge as full sexual beings. It's taken me a long time to be able to say this and, as you'll see, my use of pornography has not been at all straight-forward and has, at times, been contradictory.

I first encountered pornography at four or five when a friend and I discovered a magazine under her parents' settee. It was hardcore and I can visualize it even today. The pictures showed everyday scenes like two couples out shopping except that everyone was naked. The two couples were holding cocks and breasts the same way you'd shake hands. It would probably make me laugh now. Another showed a white woman who had kidnapped a black slave who she forced to lick her pussy until he got to enjoy it (this stuff certainly put women in control!). It confirmed what we suspected but never really knew, that the grown-ups were just as fascinated by each others' bodies as we were. (This was actually quite annoying as we saw this as our game.)

It's an unarticulated secret that many girls from about four-to-eight indulge in harmless sexual gratification until conditioned to think otherwise (I remember being severely spanked). It's not a gender preference; you just tend to get palmed off with your own sex at that tender age. Looking at the magazine, we didn't know the facts of life but we knew the pleasures of licking each others' vaginas. I don't think this early encounter with pornography was damaging as my sexual curiosity was already in motion, matched only by a concern with that other taboo, death. Old people fascinated me and if they visited my house I couldn't stop looking at their terrible ravaged faces. I wanted to scream at my Mom "How can you speak to those people!?". It was along those kind of lines that my friend and I decided to find out what you looked like after you died by cultivating a piece of chocolate in a matchbox until it went mouldy and green. To our minds this first encounter with pornography rated as much significance as the curious metamorphis of the chocolate.

After we had been caught and spanked so many times our life wasn't worth living, we forgot about sex and became prudish conformists until the onset of puberty, when you get a chance to rethink your options. Ironically, when others were trying out their first condom, I was too scared even to kiss and spent ages practising on mirrors and things. Enter my second memorable encounter with pornography. I was thirteen and laid up in bed for a week with some illness. I had taken to reading sexy bestsellers in an attempt to learn how to do it and in the middle of one particular scene suddenly felt this strange sensation Down There. It was just as if someone had taken a magic pen and painted a stripe of wetness on my vagina. When I touched myself and found I was slippery I began masturbating for the first time in years. Playing with myself proved habit-forming for a while, aided and abetted by the sex scenes in books (many of them from horror sources) although it was not matched by increased intimacy with the various boyfriends I had. Still, I did not try to buy the pornography I clearly desired, instead I would get steamy bestsellers and skim them for the significant bits and pass them round at school.

Like most teenage girls I experienced pornography second hand, watching other people's choice of video at drunken parties or checking out the magazine collections of friends' elder brothers. Unfortunately, many women never move on from this initial underage, unofficial sneak preview of pornography and the guilty feelings often accompanying such clandestine deeds. Fortunately for me, when I was fifteen my best friend, an Asian girl, used to babysit for her next door neighbour, Gayle, who was in every sense a modern woman. Vibrators of all shapes and sizes were scattered around the house which her kids played with as toys and we found the place well stocked with whisky, cigarettes, blue movies and underwear, all of which we sampled. It was "welcome to the house of sin", and once the kids were in bed we did everything we shouldn't and loved it. Gayle's brother ran a video shop and had a good under-the-counter porn line which we watched with amazement (at that time we couldn't imagine doing it). When I talked to the class film buff about the videos I was surprised to discover that you couldn't buy any of them over the counter and that he had never seen anything 'hard'. It's worth remembering that many campaigners against porn haven't, either.

I was sixteen when I finally did it, and for several years I wanted to repress my experience of all the good times had in the house of sin. It became my hidden side, the evils I had committed prior to the real inauguration with the world of flesh. My boyfriend and I were both virgins, vulnerable and eager to trade on our shared deflowering to keep the relationship together forever. Anyone or anything that threatened the shaky status quo became taboo. I had been going out with him for a year when I discovered a photo of a girl he had fancied for ages still in his wallet. We burned it. We trashed his porno magazines with their cleverly photographed girls who of course looked unimaginably more beautiful than me. We were both worried about "unwholesome" influences but because I had no porno collection, it was me who seemed to disapprove of it. He was merely terrified of the possibility of substitute vibrators and questioned my preference for certain shaped deodorant bottles and anything that might be bigger than him. Of course we both still masturbated when apart (I used to make up fantasies or remember scenes I had seen or read) and if I came across a hidden girlie magazine it confronted all those dirty secrets I was trying to hide. I hated pornography, it was degrading to women and aroused feelings of envy and shame.

Unfortunately, women are so conditioned to disapprove of or distrust any expression of female gratification that even I succumbed. There are so few women in control of their own sexuality that when you do meet them they stand out.

It wasn't until I was at University that I met Marion. I was in a dance class, had just written a play about a failed relationship and was trying to get out of my leotard and into my jeans without showing my bikini line. And there was this Scottish girl strolling around naked with willful abandon, telling me how she wanted to be a stripper. She didn't have a figure like the girls in *Knave* but she loved her body and didn't care who knew it. She regularly bought *Forum*, walked around revealing her underwear and liked to piss in public. For being like Madonna, displaying the trappings of male fantasy and parading them, she was the talk and scandal of the town. I admired her but I was still playing Miss Nice Girl, with a fiancé and a higher degree place and a life planned out. When the shit hit the fan and I ended up single, in debt and working for a corporate video company for low pay and even lower status from my male boss, it was Marion whom I turned to. Whilst she tried to launch a career in mud wrestling, I dreamed of being an editor, and our correspondence grew ever more erotic and fervent.

When you live in a dive, with no money and all your friends have moved on, fantasy becomes a big part of your life. At the place where I worked we unofficially copied porn movies to which I had free access. I also had the keys to work and could lock myself in after hours, watch whatever I liked and pleasure myself without worrying about being disturbed. It was here that I developed my own private fantasy world. As well as writing up my erotic fantasies I also began editing the porn movies to how I wanted them. Pretty soon I wanted to see how I looked in sexual postures and took topless photographs of myself by performing in front of a video and printing off stills. What I realized from my DIY porn is that your own sexual expression looks nothing like the commercial stuff available and can take any form you want it to. Just as those who buy *Cosmopolitan* don't resemble too closely the size 8 models they depict, existing and potential users of pornography don't have to look like porn models either.

Working often in a predominantly male environment my own sexual confidence means that jerks can't browbeat me on my figure and tastes because quite simply I've learnt there are more choices than just being a slut or a whore. Women are already interested in pornography but many feel too embarrassed to become consumers and take an active role in shaping the demands of the marketplace. Pornography needs to be changed so that it doesn't project only male desires. Instead of banning it, women need to participate and create pornography.

Francis Scally grew up Catholic in a sea-side village in Ireland with her seven sisters, brother and parents. The loss of her religion, which she questioned in her teens, was painful but liberating and coincided with her coming to terms with sex.

Scally has a BA Hons degree and she is taking a MA degree in Belfast exploring Renaissance society's attitudes — surprisingly similar to our own regarding sex, women, and hierarchy.

Erotique

Frances Scally

Pornography: n. writings or pictures or films etc. that are intended to stimulate erotic feelings by description or portrayal of sexual activity. Pornographic: adj.

I probably discovered pornography well before I was ten years old but if I did I can't remember any specific incidents. The first time I can actually remember recognizing porn was when I was about ten years old and I found Jackie Collins' *Hollywood Wives*. The first few pages describe incest between a young boy and his mother. It described the "warm, wet, softness" of the mother's vagina in detail and it scared me to death. I knew so little about sex and anything I did know was very basic, like seeing my older sisters kissing their boyfriends when I was supposed to be asleep and they thought they were kissing in private.

The opening chapter of *Hollywood Wives* scared me because I was reading not only about something totally new and inconceivable, but because I couldn't control it by retreating back into the safety and familiarity of my bed as usual. I *knew* something now and I also knew that I couldn't tell Mammy about it. I'd heard her saying that those books were disgusting (which ironically was probably what made me investigate them in the first place) and I wasn't even allowed in my older sister's room, where 'they' were hidden, never mind being allowed to read them.

I remember feeling a dread; I knew that I was leaving something familiar and safe behind. I ran downstairs to two of my sisters (one and two years older than me) crying (but really looking for reassurance that it wasn't true, that there was no such thing as strange and scary as sex), but one of them just laughed and said, "That's what you get for reading dirty books!" I had half expected to be dragged to the priest to be exorcized, but my sister's reaction was so healthily unmysterious it enabled me to go back a few months later and finish the book!

I didn't mention that I'd read the book to anyone else. I wanted to remain a good little girl in everyone's eyes and I knew that I would be teased if everyone knew. I would feel exposed and dirty by their reactions. This feeling is something which remained with me over the years until I eventually and painfully let go of my projected self-image as a 'good little girl'.

I read *Hollywood Wives* with guilt and fear but avidly! I spent every spare moment with my back against the door and my foot to the bed in case anyone came in unexpectedly. When anyone did come in I put the book under the bed and pretended to read *Bunty* or *Mandy* (magazines for girls) instead.

The only time I found porn threatening was when I was with a boyfriend who couldn't get sexually excited unless he was surrounded by porn. I felt a bit inadequate until I realized that he was just stuck in a rut that he was too comfortable to come out of. I eventually just found him boring and got rid of him (but I did keep his porn collection!). Porn is a means to an end; I think it shouldn't always be an end in itself (although sometimes of course it's just the thing). Variety is the spice of life and all that. . . .

I suppose porn doesn't have any conscious relevance in my life anymore insofar as I don't go out and buy it on a regular basis, although if I feel like it I do. However, I still love coming across it. I have found, however, that very little, if anything, that I read shocks me. Personally I've reached my limit as far as written pornographic fiction. Personal accounts of sexual experiences still turn me on because I suppose they're more intense and real, and they're being recounted for their own sake and not just a poor, obvious attempt at selling a magazine or whatever. I can still discriminate even when I am looking for a quick, cheap thrill and the poor quality I've encountered is the only offensive thing to me in porn. I find less obvious, more suggestive porn much more stimulating than two models in a barely awake clench. A beautifully toned muscle, a strong looking back or heavily lidded eyes, for example, does so much more for me (and female friends) than those awful poseurs wearing nothing but white socks and sun-(un)kissed white buttocks against a tan — Yuck!

Admittedly, I do find it a bit surprising how men I've known have accepted anything pornographic they've come across as potentially stimulating (although I've never been with any man with a higher sex drive than me). However, I think this is very healthy, if a trifle boring, and it may come from the fact that it is more acceptable in our society for men to be sexual, and not women. Perhaps women's seemingly more discriminating tastes are a left-over reaction to 'being nice' towards sex, even when they're sexually uninhibited in every other way.

Our society's and media's pressures are intense concerning the portrayal of women. For example, it is a standard banality to present prostitutes (who are indubitably having sex for the money) as having the inevitable 'heart of gold', as if, firstly, that indisputably sexually active women are 'bad' on the surface, rather than, more obviously, women using whatever they have; i.e., their bodies, to do business and make money for whatever reason. Secondly, even 'bad' (equated with being sexual) girls are 'good' (equated with being virginal) underneath just by virtue of being female, as if it's innate for women to only be sexual when driven by circumstances.

Feminism was supposed to be a reaction to such limiting of women's potential, but from my own experience, many women are being taught the equation that being a feminist automatically means being a censor of porn. I encountered this attitude very strongly from my peers in third-level education. People try to be 'politically correct' by denouncing pornography as supporting bad treatment of women. This is a reflection of the academic attitude (with a few exceptions) towards porn. Personally, I find it illogical and a contradiction on feminism as a by-word for women's liberation and, more sinisterly, another attempt at controlling women's sexuality, only worse because this time it comes under the name of so-called female liberation.

Porn exists in my life, but it's usually incidental. Where I've encountered it I've embraced it, sometimes defiantly, which is something I don't want. I now consciously reject being defiant about pornography as a reaction to the would-be total imposition of censorship, because I prefer to just get on with my own sex life. However, I think it is really bad that feminism is getting such a poor name because it is increasingly equated with sexual repression. Feminists are seen as unsexy, men-hating lesbians where I come from because of the bitterly vehement censorship of some feminists, like clearing the shop shelves of what they view as offensive material.

Feminism should allow each person the space to be an individual first and labeled a feminist second. The best way to contribute to a feminist movement is to lead primarily through individual example and achievement. I'm a feminist but I do not want to be neatly categorized away as such, I want to explore my personal identity, the very thing feminists accuse men of denying women and this exploration includes the expression of my individual sexuality whatever that may be. As long as I do not hurt anyone in the process then no one has the right to censor me.

I love sex and porn for me is something that is positive, a good healthy sex aid at best, repetitive and unimaginative at worst. Porn only truly offends me when it looks like someone is being exploited or hurt or definitely is not enjoying it (usually children or animals although I acknowledge their natural sexuality).

Porn is a reaction to a society which doesn't allow freedom

of sexual expression and which rejects anything but the hetero-sexual 'norm' generally. Censorship is a clue to a dangerously repressive attitude to sex. Sexual preferences are highly individualistic and personal and uniform repression can only result in even more hypocrisy and confusion and even less healthy sexual expression. Victorian London, for example, the supposed epitome of Puritanism, was rife with prostitution.

Men love my openness about enjoying sex, because so many women remain passive or subconsciously express feelings of guilt during sex. I think many women remain passive because they fear rejection for being sexual. They fear being called dirty or a bimbo because they have been conditioned to believe that being sexual is equal to having little self-respect, self-worth or intelligence. Such notions take their roots in the same fear and ignorance I felt growing up and would still be experiencing if I had not had the early influence of porn leading to the bliss of guilt-free sex.

Porn is a natural reaction to unnatural repression. Censorship is a fear of self-knowledge. Many women have been so controlled they fear being seen as being out of control, that is, uninhibitedly and boldly sexual, in case it is equated with weakness or being all those negative things we are taught about being women. Thankfully, my natural sexuality is too strong for me to try and reason myself out of it. Coming to terms with one's sexuality is difficult enough in such a screwed-up society without being forced to feel and try to relate to some sort of myth about standard sexuality and sexual practices.

Censorship of porn is not liberation, it is just someone else trying to dictate their 'norm' of sexuality deliberately ignoring the fact that we are all individuals. Ignorance via censorship may indeed be bliss but for me (carnal) knowledge empowers and helps liberate the woman from the 'good little girl'. Pornography breaks down gender assumptions and asserts the individuality which I for one demand and embrace. We must all have the unrestricted right to choose and to express ourselves sexually if ever we are to be truly liberated.

Anna Lynn Tercourse was brought up in the countryside, a wild place with rivers and mountains, but was soon sent away to a boarding school. The nuns were very strict, but Tercourse survived her convent education, married and had children. Tercourse's sexual appetites have increased and broadened with age and experience. Her partner is very sexual and they enjoy pornographic films, pictures and books; particularly S/M material. Their life together is a colourful variety of imaginary fantasies and real fantasy, sometimes with others invited in to watch or be included in the event. Tercourse just wishes she didn't have to be so discreet — it all seems perfectly normal to her.

Pornography & Me

Anna Lynn Tercourse

I was a pornographer at twelve years old.

I created my own material by drawing pictures designed to excite *me*. I was not skilled in drawing, unlike my sister and my school friend Barbara. However I drew pictures for myself which excited me, almost always with some kind of sadomasochistic theme. The subject I remember best is the one I drew of a long-haired naked woman being dragged along by her hair but there was never an image of the person pulling her. He, for it was a he, was always out of the picture. Another one was a buxom female in open-legged pose with smile. I struggled with that one because I couldn't do faces. The breasts were always fulsome as I longed and dreamed of having big breasts like Barbara. As I have never acquired fulsome breasts they have remained an enduring fantasy for 40 years, a lovely turn-on for me.

I began to explore my body, consciously, before I was 11, kneading my breast buds, hopefully, imagining dramas which involved painful excitement, and a watcher or audience of some kind. Medical fantasies were favourite as they enabled all parts of my body to be engaged in the drama. The usual scenario would be my suffering self in bed and a devoted person (lover or mother or father I think) in attendance. I would enjoy an hour of fantasy before going to sleep, warmed and content.

I acted out the S/M elements in my fantasies, when I was alone in the house, by tying myself up in a stimulating way, tightly across my (small) breasts and between my legs. There was a walk-in cupboard in the bathroom with the hot water tank and pipes, to which I could tie myself. The imaginary struggle to get free would make me feel wet and sexy. I tried to draw myself like this but couldn't get it convincing. I had regular 'torture' fantasies in bed involving sharp objects on my breasts, usually the corner of my book, and some imaginary person or persons forcing me to suffer the exquisite pain. I still don't know who or what these imaginary persons were; their gender was not always defined, nor was it important; it was my fantasy after all!

My earliest memory of masturbating to orgasm would be around 12 years old. I discovered how to 'come' and learnt how to imagine my fantasies, not necessarily acting them, as it had the same effect. At about 13 or 14, I began to experience tingling in my knickers without any stimulant that I could identify. It would happen at school while I was sitting at my desk and I could almost 'come' just sitting there. I now think I was excited by my love for one of the senior sixth formers whose body I admired on the hockey pitch. I was fascinated by the 'big girls' because they had breasts and wonderful bottoms which wobbled when they walked past in the dining hall.

Once I knew I could 'come' at will I felt very powerful in spite of the guilt attached to the whole thing because of the attitude of my mother and the nuns at the convent where I went to school. The school was into sex in a big way, but of course it was a sin and we were regularly warned against it, particularly with boys. Then one springtime, during Lent, we were given a 'retreat' at school, when we were supposed to be silent for three days, pray a lot and read holy books. The priest they brought in to run the retreat offered to hear our confessions, have private talks with us, and tried to deal with issues raised by the anonymous question box. I wouldn't even be seen near the question box in case any of the issues were traced to me. Anyway the highlight of the retreat was this priest delivering a sermon to around 300 pubescent girls about how to be clean and holy women, like Our Lady[13], who was so pure and free of sin that she was assumed bodily into heaven without having to go through the inconvenience of dying, burial and resurrection. The theme of his sermon was 'impurity' and self-abuse and what a serious sin it was. He even went so far as to suggest that the sin might be *mortal*, an important definition for us, as sins in the mortal category included murder and 'big' lies. We had been told that if we died in a state of mortal sin we would go straight to hell. After the sermon no one could discuss it because we were still on retreat until we got outside school when Barbara declared that the man was a complete fool inventing sins and putting ideas into our heads. I kept quiet because the ideas were already in my head and no one else said anything.

I found all sorts of ordinary pictures incredibly exciting, particularly something with a suggestion of violence or domination. The religious books we were given were full of gory details of saints being martyred which I found really exciting. Some old editions went in for pictures which turned me on. The sex of the 'martyr' was immaterial, it was the bodily engagement I found stimulating. Stories of the virgin saints were particularly good because they were nearly always martyred by wicked men who wanted to disgrace them by taking away their virginity. St Cecilia was a particularly sad case as her beheader wasn't quite competent and left her head half on, so she suffered a lot. St Maria Goretti was the best story, another virgin; the wicked men stripped her naked (phew I loved it!) and so that they couldn't

---

[13] Editor's note: Our Lady = Virgin Mary, for all you atheists out there!

satisfy their desire to disgrace her, God made her long hair grow rapidly to cover her entire body. What a turn on.

The pictures of St Lawrence on his bed of coals, being cooked to death (naked of course), and St Margaret being squashed to death under a door were all very exciting as well as the pictures and descriptions of the fate of other English martyrs, who were hung first, then their guts were pulled out in front of them and their bodies were pulled apart by four strong horses. Apparently these martyrdoms pulled in huge crowds so I'm not the only one who enjoyed it.

When I got involved with men I masturbated a lot for relief, as no sex was permitted in my catholic life. I got particularly desperate when I was living in a catholic hall of residence during my college years, and my boyfriend was not allowed on the premises. The Spanish religious community was very strict about men, and we would spend an hour necking and petting outside in the garden getting very excited indeed before I had to go inside at 10:30. As the bathrooms were public I couldn't get the privacy I needed and I shared a room with three other women. My orgasms were achieved under the bedclothes with a rubber hot water bottle which masturbated me beautifully and, as far as I know, without the knowledge of my roommates. My weekly or fortnightly confession in church included the sin of 'Impurity' and on one occasion the priest invited me to his private room to explain my problem. He asked me for details of what I was doing with myself and with men and I began to feel a bit funny. I left quickly and only much later realized that he was getting a turn on for himself, probably masturbating under his cassock.

Eventually I became involved with a strict catholic man, who was himself liberated by my sexual desire, and we were married. I became pregnant immediately and spent a steamy nine months in love with my burgeoning body, big breasts at last. I spent hours strutting in basques and tiny G strings to an imaginary audience.

Thereafter my sexual life was split — half with my husband having orgasms by, with and from him; the other half alone with my fantasies and orgasms-of-my-own. My next two pregnancies followed immediately, because as we were Catholics we used no contraception. My private times in the bathroom were the only pleasures in a life of continuous nappies and feeding, whilst our budget couldn't accommodate paying baby-sitters and outings. When I got some part-time work things got easier and I re-entered the real world, causing comment at work by going braless (small breasts see?) and wearing trousers (in a school!). The men on the staff were appreciative and said so, which I found exciting, especially when I told my husband about it and I now realize he liked hearing about other men admiring me.

I discovered softcore pornography through my friend Sally, who was doing a modeling job for *Mayfair*. I was determined to see her and bought a copy rather shamefully. I was instantly turned on and had an orgasm in a public toilet I got so desperate. The excitement came from the pictures of all these women strutting and posing *just like me.*

The combination of pictures, my fantasies and a brush handle (kept for the purpose) was a magic potion for me. Given privacy and space, I could treat myself to a night in or an afternoon with guaranteed excitement and pleasure. When my husband was abroad I enjoyed the empty house, walking around in sexy gear, getting turned on by the feel of tight G strings and open top bras. My private world remained private while I was married, as masturbation was never mentioned between us (it being a sin) although he did it regularly too, sometimes in bed beside me when he couldn't sleep. Later he deprived me of sex by masturbating downstairs before coming to bed and I began to feel resentful, wondering if this was all that life had to offer.

Later I was introduced to pornographic video films by my new partner. At first they just blew me away — I got excited immediately by anything. Now I like the old S/M theme to be there or some strong anal penetration, or best of all a combination of both. I just can't help imagining it's me and I'm excited. I can't watch a pornographic film without touching myself — I'd have to cross my legs and throb. I visit cinemas regularly with my partner and all the audience is men. I don't know why women aren't there. I find it both exciting and relaxing, and it's free for women. Sometimes I come during a film, as do many of the men, and this can excite the men around me. Even so, their behaviour is courteous and they do not presume to touch me although I do sometimes allow them to 'help' me by squeezing my breasts, sucking my nipples and holding my legs. I enjoy the experience of just letting go in the cinema, watching the screen with my legs apart, a man on each nipple, my partner rubbing my clitoris, and a prick in each hand if I want it. Sometimes the 'audience' gets in the way and I can't see the film!

When the show includes a stripper I do not get excited by her, although I admire what she does and respect her work. An exception was at a show in Barcelona where one of the women strutted obscenely and I still visualize her, with her bare bottom stuck out, in an open denim jacket and cowboy boots, showing huge breasts and proud of them. Lovely!

Some visual material, alongside a good S/M story like *The Story of O*, is very stimulating for me and turns me on even when I think I'm tired. A recently imported picture book version of the story in Portuguese made me very horny indeed, and picturing the images gives me a tingle in my clitoris. The combination of anal penetration and S/M activity is magic for me. My partner loves my taste in pornography and he provides regular video material, either S/M or anal, for our sessions. When we watch a film, I come and come until I'm done and then we bring him to orgasm without the film on so that we can concentrate on each other. On other occasions he talks me through stories with an anal and/or S/M theme, and my imagination and my fingers bring me to orgasm.

I realize that the S/M desire theme has been with me almost all my life and it probably always will be.

Annie Sprinkle was born Ellen Steinberg in 1954 in Philadelphia PA, USA. Her family moved to Los Angeles, then Panama. At seventeen, Sprinkle returned to the US with her boyfriend to live in an artist community. After being a full-time hippie for a year, she worked in a massage parlour only to discover she'd become a hooker which, she decided, was great, rather like being a nurse.

Sprinkle met Gerard Damiano, the director of the porno hit, Deep Throat, *who eventually brought her to New York and put her into hardcore movies. She starred in two hundred and twenty porno films in total, became a centerfold model, a character in National Lampoon's Foto Funnies, a fetish model and then started posing for more experimental lesbian photography.*

In 1978 she got involved with the publishers of LOVE, an alternative reader-written porno paper, and then met Willem de Ridder who whisked her off to Italy for a year and a half of bliss. Missing the bright lights, Sprinkle felt ambitious and returned to New York, where she was proclaimed an artist and started her experimentation with S/M, piss sex, photography and performance. Her alternative form of burlesque called Strip Speak resulted in the head of performance studies at New York University inviting her to do a show.

Sprinkle has produced a mass of charming sex positive art, poetry, articles (including "How to fuck and type at the same time"), tattoo art, tit prints, installations, performance and drawing. Her writing is never bashful, and includes the line "The porn I get most turned on watching is sex with animals." She has become politically active, joining Prostitutes of New York, going on marches and fronting rallies.

Annie has toured the world with her performances and workshops. She recently took a year's sabbatical to reassess her life and decide where she wanted to go next. Tuppy Owens interviewed her at her new home by the sea in East Hampton, New York, to find out her current views on pornography.

The Best is Yet To Come

Annie Sprinkle

I expressed my views on pornography in 1991, in my book *Annie Sprinkle, Post Porn Modernist* with the following passage to help people see that being in porno, like many other careers, has its advantages and disadvantages:

"MESSAGE FROM THE MIDDLE"

> *I've seen pornography help people, and I've seen pornography hurt people. Being in pornography has helped me and, in some ways, it may have hurt me.*
>
> *I've been exploited by pornography, and pornography has paid my bills for the past twelve years (mostly I've exploited pornography).*
>
> *I suppose pornography has caused a few rapes, and I suppose it has prevented a few. I've seen pornography help people solve some of their sexual problems, and I've seen pornography create sexual problems for others.*
>
> *While making pornography, I sometimes have felt sexually jaded and confused, and sometimes I feel very free and joyful.*
>
> *Some of the pornography I've made is pretty awful schlock, and some of the pornography I've made is very creative, interesting, wonderful stuff I'm proud of, and it's been educational and helpful to others.*
>
> *Sometimes I wonder if any of my work in pornography may have hurt the women's movement, yet mostly I feel like a women's liberation freedom fighter who is contributing some-*

thing to women's liberation (particularly women's sexual liberation), and that makes me happy.

For better or worse, I will continue to express myself with sexually explicit images, creating what I like to create, doing what I like to do, and there is no other side to this coin."

Since I wrote that, I've got a much less positive view about the porn industry. When AIDS hit, I saw how most people in the industry don't care about much except money. Like other industries, there are power struggles and there's a lot of non-caring.

I'd like to see people working towards connecting sexually, on a much deeper level, although many of us are afraid of intimacy and deep love, even though I think that's what we really want.

Hamburgers aren't very nourishing but they sell a lot of them. It's that way with porn. It's not ideal but at least it's something. But, just because something feels good and gives you an orgasm, doesn't make it really nourishing for you on a deeper level. A lot of commercial sex doesn't bring fulfillment and happiness. Many men use it outside their relationship causing dishonesty and guilt. I know that people do the best they can, but in an ideal situation, people should be honest with themselves and their partners. Now I see how a lot of pornography, S/M and paid sex can perpetuate childhood neuroses, sexual misconceptions and misogyny.

These days, I'm a lesbian, committed to making the best possible world for women. I don't want rough, hurtful sex any more, to give it or receive it. I want to be able to look into my lover's eyes and connect in a loving way. Sometimes, I think I did some things because I had a low self image. I acknowledged only the good times, and denied the rest. I've become much more honest with myself, and have a clearer idea of what I really want.

Mind you, men who use pornography can be victims of the status quo as well. It's time they grew up and got real. The problem is that many of them are totally guilt-ridden, insensitive, unaware and disrespectful of women. It's time to create a new world. Hetero porn is stuck in the garbage heap. Women are porn's new pioneers. *On Our Backs*, the San Francisco lesbian magazine, was the first magazine which dared show a very different aesthetic on what is sexy. I think Susie Bright and Debbie Sundahl really did a great service. They were amongst the first Post Porn Modernists. Most of the really interesting porn and erotica now is being done by people who were never in the porn industry. It's very hard for people in the industry to change over to something new and more interesting.

I should make it clear that I'm not against pornography. I'm just trying to improve it. I'm trying to change some of the outmoded ideas of pornography, and its limited view of what is sexy. Take silicone breasts for example. A friend of mine had three heart attacks from her silicone breasts and that freaks me out. Why? Because you make more money as a stripper if you have large breasts. I say, rather than women getting breast implants, we should change people's views. If a woman wants to jut out, she can stuff a bra.

My interest in commercial pornography has diminished because now I am more of an artist, not a supplier of goods. I want to be the person who stimulates ideas and concepts and who pushes the envelope. I share what I discover, through my work. I no longer care about pleasing the average person. I don't want to stay 'teacher in the kindergarten', or the party girl. I know this sounds elitist and classist but I want to create new things.

Things are changing and have got a lot better, especially for women. Six years ago, when I was teaching a workshop, I asked women if they knew where their G-Spot was, only two or three would raise their hand out of a group of thirty or forty women. Now, eighty percent know. "How many of you ejaculate?" At least a third of them ejaculate. They are much more aware. "How many have had an energy orgasm?" a third of them raise their hands. Women have become a lot more knowledgeable and empowered. That's a good thing. At least now most guys know where the clitoris is. Not so long ago, a lot of them didn't know. Really! Hard to believe but true. We've cum a long way, baby.

But I don't want to continue to teach people where the clitoris is, I want to teach people how to be authentic, go deeper, honestly communicate their desires. Lots of women aren't able to ask for what they want or speak the truth. I want to teach women how to expand their orgasm, enter spiritual grounds, I want to explore getting all this into museums, making sex a more prevalent subject matter in art and culture.

There's a lot more freedom. People are publishing stuff that's never been done before. Charles Gatewood and Fakir Musafar and others are supplying so much alternative input. I was recently at the Whitney Museum's Biennial Show, where they show the crème de la crème, and saw quite a bit of sex. In fact, Cathy Opie, who used to shoot for *On Our Backs*, had photographs there, and there were Mapplethorpes. It was highbrow porn, and there's lots of room for that. Then there are people like Nan Goldman, the amazing photographer who has done a lot of pictures of prostitutes and drag queens, documenting the underground sex scene. Even in religion, we're seeing more and more spiritual and religious groups incorporating sexuality. You'll see more nude beaches, a lot more awareness of abuse issues. The biggest challenge is dealing with children and sexuality because people are totally off-base with it. People don't know how to deal with it. I don't even think I'll see it taken care of in my lifetime. When I teach my workshops, women say things like, "Oh! I wish my twelve-year-old daughter could come to this," or "I wish all young women were taught sexuality this way." It's a very safe and loving way to learn. There's always this sense that girls have learnt about sexuality from their elders, but today, it's taboo.

I've finished my pin-up photography era. I'm writing articles, teaching workshops, displaying my work in art galleries, and doing my shows. My latest performance was about stripping, where I took every striptease cliché in the book and have a love/hate relationship with it, kind of like a clown. There are lots of gimmicks and props and costumes and it has a poignant ending. Also, I'm producing a computer mouse pad with my photograph on it. I'm continuing my own studies and research on sex, healing, magic, love, etc., always.

Of course, I hate censorship, and these days, I'm more willing to take risks now that I've got lawyers behind me (many of my lesbian friends are lawyers). I always avoided getting arrested before, now I'm willing to publish things I might have been afraid of. On the other hand, my stuff is less hard core, partly because I'm becoming more private. After showing my cervix to millions of people (now it's on the Internet), and having sex in front of millions of people on screen, I am experimenting with keeping my legs shut! It's kind of an adventure. I really feel that my best work is yet to come. Definitely. In this last workshop I just taught, I went further than I ever thought I could go. It was so incredible and beautiful and enlightening. The best is yet to come.

I have great optimism for the future. Sex has been so incredibly underrated, misunderstood and limited in the way it's portrayed, there's so much room for growth and improvement.

I'm lucky because I've managed to earn a living for the past three years only working for other women. My workshops, videos and photography are all made for women. I never thought this would be possible. I did love what I did before and have no regrets but I'm forty years old and smarter. I now see things for what they are. My goal is to live a pleasure-filled, comfortable ecstatic, happy, blissful, playful, sensuous, beautiful life. I'd like to make the world a more happy, playful, less violent, more sexually satisfied, more loving place. It sounds like a 1960s ideal but I see so many people unsatisfied. There is so much to learn. I have learnt, for example, how so many women are unaware cohorts of the patriarchal sex system, and so trained just to please men. Garter belts and corsets are not what we truly want. In my workshops, when the women do the Taoist erotic massage ritual, they are moved to tears. They don't cry during the Sluts rituals. Costumes are superficial. They are not deeply moving or intimate. You know, I was at the Hellfire Club in New York and had twenty guys piss on me, I was in a circle jerk. It was very interesting, I had a wet pussy, it was a turn-on, I had orgasms but it didn't move me or satisfy me the way Tantric or Taoist sex rituals do.

Although I talk about the value of deep relationships, I am still not that good at them (we do teach what we want to learn). I realise I too have fear of intimacy, fear of really being loved, even though this is what I really want.

I did enjoy being a sacred prostitute, out there giving my sexual gifts, being a promiscuous experience-seeker. I've seen relationships as traps, as prisons, and a lot of them are. After my recent three-day workshop, all the women felt loved, appreciated, accepted for who they are, and supported. We all felt really good about ourselves. We created a safe, honest, deeply satisfying environment to explore the depths of our sexualities, and we were all accepting of our differences and acknowledged our similarities. This was a group of all women, but it can happen with men too.

Our sexuality is not only something that can be used for the enhancement of an intimate relationship, for physical pleasure or procreation, but it can also be used for personal transformation and emotional healing, self-realisation and spiritual growth, and as a way to learn about all life and death. A focused, sexually awakened group is a divine and extremely powerful force that can not only inspire each person in the group, but has the potential to contribute to the well-being of life on earth as well.

Tuppy Owens was brought up in Cambridge and now lives in London. Her early life was spent working as an ecologist — then she discovered porn. Owens has written a novel about her experiences in making blue movies. The Making of Sensations *was published in 1994. As well as publishing, she organises the annual Sex Maniacs' Ball, to encourage her readers to come out and express their wildest fantasies.*

She has a Diploma in Human Sexuality from London University and an Honorary Doctorate from the Institute for the Advanced Study of Human Sexuality in San Francisco. Owens is an active member of Feminists Against Censorship and this book could never have come into being if it were not for her ideas and contacts.

An Autopornography

Tuppy Owens

I love porn very much. I love looking at it. I work in it. It is my life. Being with it all the time, it is my normal reading matter. This is my Autopornography.

It's not like, "I think I need a wank, I'll look at some porn." I'm not really into using other people's imagery for my own sexual gratification. In fact, I'm not really into fantasy much. I'm a doer, not a dreamer. I get off on being with an exciting partner, touching myself or being touched. On the rare occasions I want to think of something to get excited, it's me being eleven years old with perky tits, getting ravaged by a gang of luscious boys. I might be in the back of a car with several of them, dressed in skimpy clothing and their hands delving into my top and pants. We'd be on the way to the house where they would fuck me endlessly, each one of them finding me irresistible. If there was porn like that, I might buy it (but I think it would always be sold out — that's if it were ever allowed!). If I'd been asked to do such a movie when I was eleven, I would have jumped at the idea. But then, where would my fantasy be now? I think that I've had this fantasy since I was four years old. I remember at night, my bed became a house where the boys lived with me, and they all desired me.

Sex has always been essentially the most exciting thing in my life. As a youngster, I saw no need for special books on it, because sex should be in every book. I remember buying a copy of a tit mag when I was quite young, and thinking it was just a general interest magazine.

In my early twenties, I was extremely lucky to be introduced to hardcore pornography by a cultured man who had a fabulous collection of French and other foreign erotica. He showed me a copy of the Swedish magazine, *Private* and my eyes lit up. I thought it was wonderful. I wanted to do it, try it, be part of it. Happily, my dream came true.

He and I set up an erotic publishing company together but, due to the laws in this country, we only made softcore. I always used to think I could never do hardcore photography anyway, because I couldn't possibly focus the camera lens accurately if I was turned on, and I would be terribly turned on if I were photographing people shafting and sucking each other.

Even though my books and products have been softcore, I've acted in a couple of hardcore movies and contributed to hardcore magazines. I prefer porn to be as strong as possible. Erections are elegant. Looking at a picture of insertion is just like seeing a painting of someone coming through the garden gate after a hard day's work, with smoke coming out of the chimney of the house and you can almost smell the supper. "Oh, yes," you go, "home!". And of course, everyone wants to see a picture of a boy or girl making out with a pig at least once in their lives, then their curiosity is satisfied. It's pretty harmless, really.

When I first saw porno videos, I couldn't understand how anybody could sit watching them without jerking off, and I found the experience of being turned on in a room full of people and having to "behave" myself difficult to cope with. I still don't like being in that situation. I usually go off to make the tea! Porn images do give me an enormous amount of pleasure. I find them sexually aesthetic. I particularly like *Foreskin Quarterly* although it's very hard to get hold of. Looking at pictures of foreskins makes my mouth water.

Sometimes when I'm working with porn, I get the need for a wank. Mostly, I can't quite remember which image it was that set me off! It could be a lusty lady in American *Penthouse*. Guccione has the knack of seduction in his photography. They say he always gets the girl horny before he starts taking the photos. Amateur stuff can be exciting, too, without all that makeup and styling.

I've enjoyed watching live sex shows. I thought the people were very skilled and I like watching skilled sex. In the last show I saw, at The Baghdad in Barcelona, a very young couple in their late teens were doing some acrobatic sex and I realised that they were doing things I used to do at that age. That made me realise I should work at staying agile, because I'd totally forgotten some of my favourite sex positions.

Porno is good when you see something that impresses you, but that's rare. Porno sex is usually much less impressive than real sex. However, I do love images of people when you see signs of them being really turned on, like bodies which are flushed red, sweating, shaking, dribbling. I like it when people go completely berserk. Shame it's so rare.

I like to make a differentiation in my mind, in real sex between what I call pornographic sex and intimate sex. Porno sex is highly visual, picturesque: beautiful blow jobs, him coming over my face, me squatting over him and pissing on him, doing it on a fire escape. Part of the thrill is the scene you are projecting. Flexing your muscles or stretching your neck, or getting squirted on, creates incredible images that make you feel wonderful.

Intimate sex, on the other hand, can be just as hot, or more so, but provides none of the above. All the tension is going on between you, enclosed by your passion.

Similarly, relationships can be pornographic, when you share your wildest fantasies and plan sexual escapades. They can also be intimate, when you share your lust dreamily, and only want to hold hands, cuddle and smooch.

This distinction is relevant to an essay on pornography, because porn has influenced human behaviour. Thanks to pornography, people enjoy more adventurous sex. Twenty years ago, I've been told by a friend from Dubai, most Arab couples in the Gulf had sex in bed at night, with the lights off. They are traditionally extremely private and rather sexually reserved. Nowadays, with porno videos dubbed into Arabic and circulated around secretly, many Arabs are enjoying the type of sex they see in blue movies, like oral sex on the floor in the light. This must be true for many couples around the world — porno peels the bed covers back.

Of all the porno videos I've ever watched, I think my favourite is a "silent movie" vintage compilation called *What Got Grandpa Hot*. There's something about the sex in these films that they can't seem to manage to portray anymore: it's coy, witty, hot and natural. They frig each other with fast-moving hands, kiss with open mouths as if they can't get enough, and they came in all shapes and sizes. It makes today's porn, with its shaved pubes and silicone tits, seem so sterile.

I can't be arsed to read much erotic fiction. Nobody has ever come close to Henry Miller for me. He wrote erotic passages like "In the blind hole of sex she waltzed like a trained mouse, her jaws unhinged like a snake's, her skin horripilating in barbed plumes. She had the insatiable lust of a unicorn, the itch that laid the Egyptians low."

For a man who declared, "I want a world where the vagina is represented by a crude, honest slit," he didn't half make cunts sound great: "It was an enormous cunt too, when I think back on it. A dark, subterranean labyrinth fitted up with divans and cosy corners and rubber teeth and syringes and soft nettles and eiderdown and mulberry leaves." Before Betty Dodson came along, he was the cunt saviour. I didn't want to wank over Miller, just read, and feel like you do when you're in the middle of a long hot fuck and never want to come. Desired, caught up in it, hungry for more. This is what I want porn for. When people talk about "using porn" I cringe a little. It's like buying a picture to cover up the stain on the wall. Getting turned on to come during wanking is fine but orgasm is not the be-all and end-all in sex. Nobody ever talks about the quality of the journey, just getting there. We certainly have got a long way to go!

You may be surprised that I used the word "desired"; porno is about making you feel desire — how can it make you feel desired? I remember the manageress of The Cheetah Lounge explaining on a recent TV show about lap dancing, "If you really want to earn a lot of money, act like a lady. What you have to do is make the guy want you. Then he will wink at his friends and say 'That girl really wants me'." She made me realise how very much one has a relationship with porn, gets wrapped up in it, taken with it, so you feel wanted. This is why I've never been able to understand why most porn is made to be so unaffectionate towards the reader/viewer. Perhaps punters want to keep the image of those "people with perfect bodies" as out of reach, unobtainable, but that doesn't mean the whole magazine or film has to feel icy cold.

Porn, for me, should be created with love. The only thing I've ever taken to bed with the attitude that I'm bound to end up tossing off is the little reader-written, photocopied black and white, sexzine called *ApaEros*. All the subscribers get the chance to contribute and nothing gets censored. I love feeling there's this little family of people all over the world, getting each other hot and horny for fun.

Gay porn has always been a big turn on for me. Some of the stories in the lesbian magazine, *Quim* have been provocative and I get all steamed up over the all-male volumes like *Wads* and *Juice* which are true experiences from *STH: The New York Review of Cocksucking.*

Apart from this, Carol A. Queen and David Aaron Clark are perhaps the best contemporary porn fiction writers, approaching my Henry Miller ideal. I nominated them both for the 1994 Erotic Oscars, which was the first of what I hope might be an annual celebration of the best pornography and erotic efforts. It's always been my aim to strive for improvement, encourage people with talent, to make porn better and to help people get more out of it. It was interesting that the judges had a hard time agreeing but then, you couldn't hope to find a more diverse bunch of people if you tried. We realised that there is no "best", as it depends on your mood and situation. Sometimes porn needs to be sleazy and sometimes it needs to be sophisticated, sometimes you want it blatant, sometimes subtle.

The most expensive porn I ever bought was a French antiquarian book which cost £400! I do absolutely love it and treasure it but really hate owning anything that valuable. It contains the most adorable water colours, of people in the country screwing and licking each other, romping rudely over hillsides, in boats and in the hedgerows. The pricks and tongues are very rude red. I suppose it was the screwing in the punt that made me buy it. I love sex by the water. My ambition for my old age is to write the porno version of *Wind in the Willows*.

People often ask me if working in porn makes me jaded. The answer is no. I might get fed up with packaging things up for mail order, doing VAT returns and chasing unpaid invoices, but the sex is always great. You can never know it all — each piece of knowledge opens up new doors and leads to more fun and excitement. I love working and living amongst a sea of porn. Men who've lived with me have sometimes found it a bit overwhelming, but that's their problem.

I've only ever "caught" two boyfriends with porno and, both times, it was a bit of a shock. The first was when we were on holiday, and I realised that he was spending an awful lot of time with the super 8 movie camera we'd borrowed, standing at the side of a field, shooting the horse's erections. Back home, our holiday film swung across the wall in the form of endless black dongs. I must say, I roared with laughter and was pleased he'd found a new hobby.

The second time, I woke up and realised that my "then" boyfriend wasn't in the bed, and went in search of him. He was in the bathroom, jerking off over a magazine. He was bent over the wash basin with his dick pointed down into bowl, pulling at it, looking at the magazine which was propped up on the basin. It was one of my very old porno mags from the 50s, with only nude men in it.

I thought this might be a bit more serious. I told him that if he liked men, he should fuck one, but he refused to discuss it. I felt I had discovered something he was horribly ashamed of, an ugly homophobic aspect linked to his problem with women, me in particular. I was absolutely unable to see the funny side of it, unlike the horses. It made me feel bad.

The difference between these two occasions was enormous. The first boyfriend was open, the second furtive. The first experience was a laugh, the second was horrific.

But it showed me how important porno is — both times, the medium was supplying something that I could never supply myself, not being a horse nor a man. How great that people have this really safe outlet for desires that cannot be satisfied by the one they love!

I've hardly ever "used" porno in a relationship except with the man who I caught jerking off over the male naturist mag (surprise, surprise!). He wasn't all that enthusiastic about fucking me, and I would put a porn video on the VCR for him to look at while I sucked his cock. I would get turned on and forget all the problems we had, and just enjoy sucking and fucking his huge dick. It wasn't all that sad because he did love me.

Obviously my family knows what I do and it's cool with them. One of my brothers is a vicar and we once jokingly agreed that he would write some religious porn for me and I'd write some horny epistles for him. My youngest brother was in hospital for a long time in his early teens and asked me to bring him a blow-up doll, which I did, and he used her. I sent copies of *Big Ones* to my father and brought him the latest editions when he was on his death bed in hospital. My mother sometimes uses my *Planet Sex Diary* but covers up the sex positions when referring to it while out. She wasn't too happy when she got raided by some ridiculous squad of over-zealous cops who decided I was using her house as a hardcore porn hideout! Perhaps some distant relatives disapprove but they don't show it.

There are aspects of porno that I don't like. I don't like the fact that there is so much ripping off, people falling for the same old ads, that promise what will never be supplied. I also hate the fact that porn, at its most soulless, top shelf moronic state, is all there is for some men.

A male member of Outsiders (a self-help group I founded some time ago, for people isolated by physical and social disability) wrote the following to me, in one of his blacker and more lonely periods.

> *"Most sex-positive people are so anxious to close ranks against the Dworkin/Mackinnon mafia that they're reluctant to acknowledge the dark side of porn. This is one area where the voice of the dedicated consumer is rarely heard: the pornographers and libertarians slug it out with the Jesus freaks and feminists, and no-one seems particularly interested in what the wankers who buy the stuff feel. Everyone's pursuing their own agendas and vested interests, and finding out how things actually are, clearly isn't a priority.*

> *"One reason why my taste for porn is giving me particular grief at the moment is that it's exactly ten years since I fell into the trap. Before then, I could take it or leave it, but in the past seven or eight years, I've bought at least 2,000 magazines, all thrown away soon afterwards in a spasm of self-reproach.... Porn is a sweet but temporary escape from the*

*loneliness brought on by my stammer. . . . I'm desperate to
find a more sharing way of being sexual."*

I remember putting his letter down on the table and feeling cold. He's left out in the cold, resigned to his isolation, and
feeling that wanking over a photo is the nearest he'll come to an
intimate relationship with a woman.

The addiction doctors would say that this man is addicted
to porn, but I would say that he is a healthy individual living in
a sick society. He's got a wonderful sex drive, just waiting for a
woman to make the most of. But since most women turn their
noses up at rampant men with stutters, oops! there goes another
precious erection, spunk all over the pretty face in the picture in
the magazine!

After being involved in Outsiders for fifteen years, I know
one thing. Being disabled normally makes it even more difficult
than usual to find the right partner and, on the whole, in the
heterosexual world anyway, it is far more difficult for disabled
men. This is because men are more accepting of disability in a
partner than women are. Even though lots of men talk about
wanting 'good looking girls with perfect bodies', all women are
wanted by them for friendship, sex and marriage, whatever their
appearance, and despite problems such as stammers. On the
other hand, women tend to be much fussier, presumably, it
seems, because we tend to have a lower sex drive and, of course,
we can afford to be fussy, since so many men desire us. What
women seem to want is a man who is pleasing to look at, who
can talk, walk and fuck. A male with a stammer, as I said, is an
embarrassment.

I have almost become the editor of several of the new sex
magazines for women/couples. There have been about eight of
them in Britain and they attracted a whole load of publicity. At
last women could look at men the way men have always looked
at women. But they were never erotic. They offered women
consolation, information, gay imagery, but never titillation,

romance or fun. My efforts to improve this obviously terrified the publishers so much that I never got the chance to actually go ahead. I wanted to make enormous changes. Erotic magazines for women should take pride in female sexuality, and stop copying the men's sex mags and the women's fashions mags. The dummies of my two proposed sex mags for women, *Hausfrau* (1984) and *Shady Madonnas* (1993) sit here, gathering dust.

I feel porn mags should stop being slick and start being sexy. Sexy is pretty, messy, vulgar, hot, funny and smoochy. Personal and mysterious, hairy and smooth. Fat and thin. Fleshy and clothed.

Mind you, it's pushing shit up a hill in Britain, because we're censored at every corner. Printers, distributors, shopkeepers, local busybodies, all try to stop us. The distributors are the biggest censors. As a publisher, you get so frustrated you just want to put rude pictures inside windows, like an advent calendar. That way, the poor little delivery man and newsagent won't have to know he's selling pictures of cocks in gobs and up bum holes.

Sadly, the cutting tool for the "advent calendar porn" would be horribly expensive. Anyway, everyone would peep, and then the windows wouldn't close properly and I would have to go to prison. Back to the drawing board!

Sometimes I wonder if the reason why we British have such strong censorship laws isn't anything to do with sex, but it's about money. We are extremely puritanical about money. We always find it shocking when we hear foreigners discussing money, because we never do. Perhaps it's the selling of sex we cannot stand. After all, we're a pretty rampant nation, most of us enjoy sex to the full, once we find the right partner. So, maybe prostitution and pornography are unacceptable here only because they have to be paid for.

Well, girls, time to start giving it away!

Lucy Williams was born in July 1969 and at the age of ten moved to a village called Misterton in Somerset, England, where she lived for nine years. During her time in Misterton she suffered and recovered from anorexia and a nervous breakdown. After a two year art foundation course, Williams moved to Brighton and began studying for her degree in 3D design.

Williams left the course, finding it too restrictive, and got involved with the "Traveller" community and supporting travelling as a valid choice for a way of life. This led to being chased by the police from county to county until she finally settled in London.

Now settled, she creates collages and has had some poems published. Williams has started a degree course in Media Studies, and had two exhibitions of her recent work. One exhibition received several complaints due to its pornographic collages and a framed used tampon.

Blood Witch

Lucy Williams

I used to hate pornography. I felt it was degrading, not only to the women who were in it but also to the men who used it. It was a man's world — a world I felt I had no part in. A closed door and a sinister one at that, I had no access. Sex was a closed subject in my family; although we are not religious, pornography was taboo. If pornography was brought up in discussion, it was seen as exploitative and degrading to women and the men that used it were perverts.

As my own sexuality grew and I started to explore my own sexual world, I felt even less connected with pornography. All the men I knew had used it at one stage or other, but none of the women I knew had even looked through a porn mag, myself included. The thought of pornography made me feel angry, reactionary towards the stereotyped, degrading images men were being fed of women. Those women were just unintelligent and weak. I felt strongly that they were the 'enemy'. The best place for pornography was for it to be banned. I felt it was doing nothing for the way men treated women, if anything it was making relations worse, and it was dangerous. Looking up at the top shelf made me feel intimidated; if I saw a man buying a porn mag I'd give him verbal hell, make him feel as uncomfortable as I was feeling. Pornography had nothing to offer me — it had no part to play in my life, I didn't want to be faced with it or have to deal with it.

Pornography wasn't for my eyes, it was for men's and I grew up with that conditioning. We live in a man's world after all, and pornography typified this feeling in me. My mother hated it, my sister hated it, all the women I knew hated it. I hated it, but deep deep down I was extremely curious, I wanted to go through the closed door, enter into the 'man's world'. Something I would never admit to myself, but it was there all the same.

At the age of twenty one I had an affair with a man ten years older than me. By this stage I felt I was a liberated woman. Sexually I was very confident and had no trouble expressing myself. After losing my virginity at the age of sixteen, I had had many lovers and two serious relationships. I knew I could relate to men, in fact I got on better with men than I did women. But the affair with the man ten years older than me was a major turning point with regard to my attitude towards pornography. He was someone very intelligent and confident and we'd spend hours talking about sex, turning each other on. He opened up very quickly to me and told me of his desire to be dominated by women, his love of stilettos, leather and pornography. He openly admitted he was a pervert and I was fascinated by him. I respected him, his views, his personality, and he respected mine — he trusted me enough to show me his collection of porn, mainly the fetish mag *Skin Two* . I loved them because they used men just as much as women, the leather and the rubber, and the freedom of expression. I didn't find them offensive at all, but very exciting. Here was someone I respected greatly and he used porn, which put me in a dilemma — I had to start rethinking my views, my own attitudes and responses. There was a side of me that still hated it, but deep down I felt I was entering the closed door, the other world.

I am now twenty five and my attitude towards pornography has changed drastically. Contrary to any conditioning, pornography is for women just as much as it is for men. Women must embrace this and realise the potential they have. We are extremely sexual, powerful creatures, we must take control of our sexuality and express it as much as possible. Celebrate — open up — it is up to us to break that damaging conditioning.

It wasn't easy for me to come to terms with pornography, there's still elements about it that I don't agree with. But there's a lot about pornography that's excellent, it's exciting and can be powerful. Not only has it helped me to express my confidence and sexuality even more, but it has helped me with my relationships with other women. I am now more in tune with the woman in me. This has developed hand in hand with my obsession with breaking other taboos, especially the taboo of menstruation. Women must rise up from feeling ashamed of their bodies: for example, the fact they menstruate. It's something to celebrate, to express and most of all to enjoy. Pornography doesn't have to be a dirty, uncomfortable word.

Two years ago I started to create collages using pornography, turning the stereotyped images of women you find in mainstream porn mags into powerful, unashamed images of female sexuality. This was quite a daunting prospect at first, but I wanted to grab pornography by the throat and give it a good kick up the arse, empowering not only the women in the mags but also myself. Sometimes, whilst looking through porn, the old feelings would creep back, but this was because I was entering into an unfamiliar world. But my responses also surprised me, I found myself getting aroused by porn, enjoying porn. It was also interesting to see how varied women's bodies were, especially when it came to their cunts — an education in itself. Obviously I knew what mine looked like, but I had never really seen what other women's cunts looked like. How unique each one is, how beautiful and most of all how powerful. Using pornography in this way has helped me enormously. My collages are a celebration and express other aspects of women's sexuality which aren't at the moment utilised in porn.

I am against censorship; I think pornography isn't honest or explicit enough. I think it should come out from under the counter, down from the top shelf and be available to all. We should show erect penises, we should show women menstruating, we should show older generations' sexuality, and disabled people's sexuality, to name a few. More women should be behind the camera as well as in front of it, and more men should be in front of the camera as well as behind it. Women as well as men should be in control of the porn industry. We are all sexual creatures. Sex is natural; it isn't dirty, it isn't something to be ashamed of. We should be celebrating it — the more open we are about our bodies and the different functions they can perform, the less sexually fucked up people there will be. We must liberate ourselves from conditioning, and from years and years of religious oppression, not just women but men also. We've all been oppressed. There's a lot that has to be changed, but I'm an optimist, it's not impossible. The new sexual, anarchistic revolution is just around the corner and it is up to us to grab it by the throat and kick it up the arse!

Nettie Pollard was involved in the Anti-Vietnam war campaign in the '60s. She was also active in the original Gay Liberation Front, the 'Women On Ireland' group, the editorial collective of the Socialist Feminist theoretical journal Red Rag, *and currently supports Spirit of Stonewall.*

Pollard has worked for over two decades for Liberty — The National Council for Civil Liberties in England. However, her most major achievement, as far as this book is concerned, is that she is also a founder member of Feminists Against Censorship.

Sexual Fantasy & Sexual Politics

Nettie Pollard

Sexual fantasies and dreams are an element in nearly everyone's life. There has been debate in the feminist movement as to the role of sexual fantasy and its possible influence on behaviour outside of the sexual context. The three theories are:

1. that certain sexual fantasy is a cause of sexist behaviour by men and an expression of self-oppression in women;

2. that sexual fantasies can be an expression and reflection of sexism in society; and

3. that sexual fantasies, whether or not you believe they are rooted in upbringing and the sexual repression of society, stand outside the ambit of sexism. This theory sees fantasy as separate from social practice.

The argument that the feminist anti-porn lobby uses against pornography is that it can influence men's behaviour outside of the sexual arena and can lead to sex discrimination, misogyny, and even rape. Many feminists who are not persuaded by this logic nevertheless feel concerned that certain types of sexual fantasy may contribute to women's oppression, and therefore see it as the task of feminists to criticize our own and other women's fantasies in order to bring them in line with our feminist politics. Women should also try to make men "clean up" their fantasies, in the same way as anti-porn women feel men should be educated not to want porn.

There is, of course, a link between the role of pornography and the role of fantasy in our sexualities. The role of pornography is to stimulate our imagination and thereby create fantasies. Pornography is not an end in itself, it's a tool.

Some feminists assert that fantasy has a direct effect on women's social, economic, political and sexual position in society. Sheila Jeffreys, author of *Anti-Climax*, states that under male supremacy, if one wonders why women are not free, one only has to look at their masochistic fantasies. She believes women should try to change and purify their fantasies in conjunction with trying to eliminate pornography. This done, men would have less stimulation for fantasies that are not "premised on equality."

The Campaign Against Pornography and Censorship (CPC) actually defines "erotica" (acceptable) as "sexual material premised on equality" as opposed to "pornography" (degrading, dangerous) which depicts power relations in sex.

Perhaps the current obsession with "cleaning up" sexual material, changing our fantasies and viewing certain expressions of sexuality as contributing to women's oppression (S/M is the current favourite) is simply a manifestation of sexual repression rather than being part of the struggle for women's freedom. Maybe seeing fantasy and, indeed, our sexual practice as a simple reflection of attitudes and practice in the world outside is not correct.

The anti-porn/anti-sex lobby make this simple equation: men who fantasize about rape go on to commit rape; therefore, they must change their fantasies, and we must remove pornography because it stimulates fantasy. But is this correct?

Do women really have more to fear from men who have rape fantasies than from those who do not? It is worth noting that, contrary to popular myth, pornography rarely depicts rape, whereas horror films, the general media and news reports increasingly feature this topic. If fantasy is so closely related to behaviour outside sexual relationships, what about the fact that women have fantasies about being raped? It is not suggested that women who have these fantasies then go out to try and get raped. There is a vast difference between what we may find stimulating in fantasy and what we may really want to do. Sex play involving rape fantasies for the purposes of arousal is probably more prevalent than is generally admitted, because it is such a taboo subject — especially amongst feminists.

And what about men? If men's sexual fantasies are simply a reflection — or worse, a cause — of sexist behaviour, then it is very hard to explain masochism and masochistic fantasy in men. It is well established that men who enjoy being beaten, humiliated or infantilized are sometimes judges, MPs[14], police officers, business executives, and others in authority in society. In fact, sexuality and position in society can be opposites.

Fantasy is the shadowy side to our sexual nature, and there is still very little known about why certain things turn us on. For instance, do rape and masochistic fantasies in women arise from women's internalization and sexualization of our subordinate role in society and in relationships, as anti-porn feminists argue? Or is the role of fantasy a little more complex? Perhaps it is not the origin but rather how we relate to our fantasies that is important.

I would argue that, while many women have fantasies that they feel guilty about, fantasy is a personal rather than political issue, and the problem is the guilt, not the fantasy. It is the guilt which should be tackled. For instance, a socially assertive, sexually confident woman challenges sexist assumptions about women by her actions and attitudes. If she has "unliberated"

---

[14] MP = Member of British Parliament

sexual fantasies, how can this affect anything outside herself and anyone she chooses to share them with? As long as she feels comfortable with her fantasies, what harm are they doing and what business is it of anyone else's?

This is true of men. too. What difference does fantasy or consensual sexual practice make except to those involved? It is rightly argued that sometimes men try to force their unwilling partners to share or act out their fantasies — the Meese Commission[15] was impressed by testimony to this effect. But the issue here is not fantasy, but rotten, unequal relationships without respect for women's sexual independence — just like rape in marriage. It is the power relations that need to change, not the fantasies.

My own view is that it may be interesting to ponder the origin and nature of our fantasies and whether we want to change them, expand them or are happy with what they are; as far as the fight against sexism is concerned, this issue is worse than a red herring — concentration on the purification of our fantasies poses a real threat to a woman's right to explore her sexuality without guilt and restriction.

We are now in the age of 'returning to Victorian values', the AIDS scare, the growing censorship of sexual materials, restrictions on sex education, and we still have Section 28[16] in force. This is the time to defend sexual diversity and the role of sexual fantasy in our lives, and not to play into the hands of the right and the anti-porn lobby by trying to restrict fantasy to what the feminist police deem acceptable.

---

[15]Meese Commission was the right-wing US Attorney General's commission on pornography under the Reagan administration. It promoted censorship.

[16]Section 28 is contained in the English Local Government Act 1988 and prohibits 'intentional promotion of homosexuality' by local authorities and the portrayal in schools of 'homosexuality as a pretended family relationship'.

Val Langmuir, a longtime activist for feminist and sexual minority causes, has been an active member of FAC since 1991. She's been a campaigner in Countdown on Spanner since 1994 and a member of the National Leather Association: International. Langmuir is against all censorship and exclusion; she spoke on behalf of FAC in the Spirit of Stonewall campaign of 1994 for the right of NAMBLA (North American Man-Boy Love Association) to march in Stonewall 25. She lives in London with a computer and doesn't know how she lived before email.

Pansexual

Val Langmuir

I'm 35 years old, identifying as a pansexual, dyke-identified, mainly submissive sadomasochist. I've been using pornography for more than 20 years now. I use it when masturbating, as an aid to fantasy when my own are getting stale (or my imagination runs out), to learn and get ideas, or just for variety. My use of it has not changed much since I first looked at it, but the material I use has become more diverse, due to the greater variety available to me now.

Although I sometimes look at videos (hardcore, mainly heterosexual), they form a small proportion of the porn I use. My preferred medium is the written word, written in the first person, where the narrator is someone with whom I can identify in fantasy. Photographs do not assist at all — they merely serve to confuse my own mental picture and detract from the fantasy. However, interestingly, drawings and particularly comic strips work exceedingly well, and these do not need to be explicit, but merely to provide a jumping-off point for my own fantasy.

I discovered porn at around the same time I first started masturbating, at about 14. I don't remember how I found out about it, but suspect that my boyfriend, who was quite a lot older than I was, must have mentioned *Forum* magazine to me — it's the sort of thing he'd have talked about, to impress me with his worldliness (it worked every time). I remember that I used to go into the newsagent's around the corner from my house and furtively buy a copy. He didn't bat an eyelid, but just put it in a brown paper bag for me. I went back around the corner, shut myself in my bedroom and began to read.

I quickly found the parts of the magazine that worked — the readers' letters. Of course there was an occasional feature article that I found arousing, but the only reliable way to get the desired result was to read those letters. And when I found one that really worked I'd read it over and over.

Later I discovered other small-format books of readers' letters culled from *Knave* and *Fiesta*. These were a bargain as they were filled with exactly the sort of thing I wanted to read, with no articles or news taking up the pages. I gradually built up a medium-sized library!

Luckily for me, the letters in these magazines often followed one of several set patterns. There were a few of these storylines that worked particularly well for me. Like the vast majority of the material in these magazines, they were heterosexual, and they were always from the woman's point of view.

One such storyline was the writer's account of how she had lost her virginity. Sometimes this involved a soldier boyfriend on leave, hitched up skirts, and knee-tremblers up against a tree, down an alley or behind a shed; other times she was working or holidaying, or evacuated during the war, on a farm, and ended up in the hay loft with a farm labourer.

Another favourite was the coercion scenario. The writer would describe how she had ended up having to have sex unwillingly. The sex had in the end been enjoyable, but she hadn't had any choice in the matter. For example, a man had taken her out to dinner, got her a little tiddly, and before she knew what was happening he had her knickers off. Or a man had picked her up hitchhiking, driven her down a dark country lane and then persuaded her that it would be better to have sex with him than to find her own way home. Or perhaps a burglar entered her house, discovered her, and decided that she was a far better prize than the TV. Or perhaps she was at an audition, or a job interview (I need not explain further).

Another storyline I liked was where the writer's boyfriend invited a gang of his friends over (perhaps his football team), and they all had sex with her. Sometimes this scenario was combined with coercion for an even more exciting story.

I used what I read as a jumping-off point for my fantasies of being made to submit by my imaginary master(s). My own fantasies were much stronger than what I read, and often featured gang-rape, beating and torture as well as the milder fantasies spawned by the porn.

Readers' letters were the mainstay of my fantasy fodder for more than 10 years. During the 80s I read *The Story of O* and *9 1/2 Weeks* and they provided additional material, which supplemented the letters; writing this I am amazed that I still did not identify as a sadomasochist at that time.

Then in 1989 a friend lent me Pat Califia's *Macho Sluts*, a collection of lesbian S/M (sadomasochist) short stories. This book changed my life. As a direct result of (but two years after) reading it, I came out as a sadomasochist, and began to have a much more fulfilling sex life, as a result of which I spent less time masturbating. At the same time I found more and more pornography to read, both more lesbian S/M material by Pat Califia and other dykes, and gay male stuff by John Preston amongst others. I became insatiable, scouring gay and alternative bookstores for any such material I could find. I began to use porn more as a tool for education than as a mere aid to fantasy. In other words I did not always masturbate when reading it, but also spent time thinking about S/M headspace and fantasy roles, and thinking about the things I read that I might want to re-enact in S/M scenes (i.e. S/M sex sessions).

Now I still read S/M porn stories, and sometimes I use them directly as fantasy material. More often though, my masturbation fantasies are reenactments of particularly exciting S/M scenes in which I have participated.

There is one more area of my fantasy that I am reluctant to mention, because I know of the prejudice it arouses. But I am writing an honest account of my sexual fantasy and of the porn that I use, so I am including it in this essay. This area is the area of man-boy sex.

In my man-boy fantasies I identify as the boy, pubescent or teen. The other party or parties might be older boys or a single adult male. Unlike my fantasies where I am a girl or woman, these don't usually include rape. They are more likely to include initiation rites as the form of coercion, for example in school fantasies. The fantasy where an adult male is involved usually involves a master/apprentice relationship.

The Batman comic has been porn for me: I've fantasised for many years about Batman and Robin as lovers. The fantasies I've had using this "porn" have consisted of myself as Robin, being a sexual object for Batman's pleasure as part of my apprenticeship to him. Boys' school stories can spark off a fantasy, especially if they contain tales of fagging or other power games; I was particularly turned on by reading "Tom Brown's Schooldays". Because of what is available it is fortunate that I don't need the story to be sexually explicit — as long as it sparks my imagination, it has done its job.

In this essay I have concentrated on describing the porn I use. But to close I'd like to make the point that porn, and my use of it, has helped me to explore my fantasies, enjoy masturbating and having orgasms, and develop my sexuality in a way that is safe and enjoyable for me. And whatever anyone may think about the porn and fantasies I have described, we should remember that porn is about fantasy. Just as I enjoy the depiction of violence in my S/M scenes, I am excited by the depiction of rape, coercion, power inequalities and plain old hot sex that I read (or imagine) in porn. This does not mean that I support real violence, rape, inequality and so on. I know the difference between fantasy and reality, between the depiction of an act and the act itself. Porn has not changed my sexuality but has merely helped to provide a channel for it. It has not made me do anything unsafe or non-consensual. It helps me to enjoy the fantasy where the reality would be distasteful, nasty, unacceptable, criminal or even impossible.

Long live fantasy! Long live pornography!

Georgina Haynes lives in London and works for various fetish publications.

Self Portrait

Georgina Haynes

Sex was always a vital part of my life long before I tried it. As a child I would be stirred by the love/sex scenes in the movies. One of my sisters and I would act them out in my room. Sexual imagery captivated me and stories such as *Angelique and the Sultan,* in which the heroine, dressed in corsets, etc., would be captured by pirates and delivered to the Sultan's harem to become the "Favourite", would take my imagination on a roller coaster ride of excitement. Strangely, I never discovered masturbation, it just didn't occur to me to touch myself. Instead I would remove my underpants and hold the gusset to my nose — I loved the smell — while I sucked my thumb (I sucked my thumb until I was 13 years old) till I fell into a dream filled sleep. These dreams would most often take the shape of many, many bodies writhing and entwining together, all shades of red, and sounds of sighing and breathing.

When I was 8 years old I used to read the newspaper to my mother who was temporarily blind and one day there was a story about a rape. I asked her what rape was and she told me. That was my first description/explanation of the sexual act. I found it very stimulating as well as thought provoking, also scary.

When I changed schools at 13 I met a gorgeous boy: Michael, my first boyfriend. First we just teased each other verbally. You know, things like — "I bet you're still a virgin" to protests of "No I'm not" to chasing each other round the playground and then actually catching each other. Believe it or not, for the first year we never kissed or petted — just shy I suppose.

He started to visit me at my home 13 miles from his and stayed longer and longer each time.

At 14 years old I had my first proper kiss, in my small attic room standing by the window with the only light from from the moon. It was mind-blowingly horny (I now know); we fell onto the bed kissing and scratching each other (I don't remember him touching my fanny[17] and I certainly didn't touch his dick). We just carried on like that for a long time, months in fact.

I knew it was inevitable we would have sex. At 15 I went on the pill with this specific aim in mind, but I had never told him I was a virgin after all nor he, me. So, I seduced my sister's boyfriend of 23. I was drunk, he put it in, he came. I thought I knew it all then so on a prearranged evening we were allowed to spend the night together in my mother's bed. Disaster! I didn't know what to do and neither did he. Oh God! So embarrassing. I didn't know you had to touch his dick or anything. It didn't happen. I left school and never saw him again. Sad, I wish I could show him what I now know.

Needless to say, that was not the end of my sex life, in fact it was quite the opposite. If somebody fancied me and I liked them, I fucked them. I was on the rampage. Between the ages of 15-27 (I'm now 38), I fucked about 100 men, no women, never wanked, and never came. I loved sex, adored men and couldn't get enough of either. In all these men there were only 2 that stood out from the rest. One, because he had a massive dick, 10 inches at least, and one because he talked dirty, pinned me down, and fucked me SO HARD I thought I'd died and gone to heaven. I fucked him on and off from 21-36.

At 27 I was single and in Amsterdam on my own for 4 weeks. One day, I went to see the movie *Cat People* starring Nastasia Kinski and Malcolm MacDowell, smoked a pipe of shit-hot weed and watched the movie. I loved that film. When I came out I thought I was a cat person. I wandered over to Leidseplein and got talking to

---

[17] English slang for pussy.

a guy, he gave me a few lines of coke but I went home on my own, aware I was very horny. I had a candlelit bath, dressed up in a beautiful regency period pink and blue lace top and played Prince very loud. I took a fairly large mirror into the bedroom — a white room with a white 4 poster bed, white lace drapes and pink satin duvet cover — and played with my fanny while looking in the mirror. I was soaking wet. I stroked and touched myself and found my clit (new discovery) and with images of the bondage and sex scenes from *Cat People* playing in my mind, I had my first orgasm. It was like an earthquake. My body was wracked. I could see my pussy spasming. Just incredible! Then I knew what I'd been missing.

In the next five years I set up my own business and had a baby (still single) but I had no more orgasms. No shortage of lovers, though. Then I met up with my on and off lover. We started to play mild S/M games — more like tie and tease really— and played with anal stimulation. I loved this. He would put his finger inside my arsehole when I was on top and talk to me about some guy coming up behind me and shoving his dick up my bum and guess what — I came again. Age 32, now.

It wasn't long before he was fucking me up the bum, tying me up, fucking my face, spunking on me and in me, telling me what a slut cunt whore I was, how he was going to put me on the street (I lived in a red light district) with my cunt exposed and a sign saying "Cunt Arsehole Blowjob Free Fuck Treat Me Rough". Come? I couldn't stop! Fab! I had discovered sex! I now found all I had to do to make myself come was to run some of these fantasies or, indeed, real scenarios through my head while playing gently with my clit. It seemed like a miracle.

When I was on a visit to him in London, he played me a porn video where two guys fucked the woman arse and cunt. When the second guy entered her my lover threw me over a stool and shoved his quite sizeable dick up my bum. My interest in hardcore porn was born. I discovered I had a voracious appetite for all forms, i.e. photographic, art, video and shortly after this first experience, cartoon porn and written stories.

I am single now and have a few fuck-buddies — single men and women, as well as couples and the odd one or four night stands. I have an extensive collection of all forms of porn, beginning to grow so much now that I'm beginning to wonder who to leave it to in my will. I had a five year relationship till summer of 94 in which we got very deep into the Fetish/S/M scene. To me it was like running around a giant toy shop and being able to choose any toy I wanted. I tried swinging — four in one night, escort work — straight, sub, and dom at £250 — £900 for four hours max, behaving like a slut in full view and often participation of many others. The fantasies grew and grew, the one-to-one scenes got more intense and serious and my orgasms never stopped. I've even been able to act out a rape by monster fantasy on stage with an audience of 3,000 people to resounding cheers and applause. What a high!

When I'm on my own feeling horny, what I will often do is start reading something such as *The Surprise Party* (a short story from *Macho Sluts* by Pat Califia) then move onto cartoon porn — more imaginative therefore much wilder than photographic or video (although I do use videos) — and look at images of gang rape, monsters raping fairies, women fucking every guy they come across, and lots of violent sex. When I feel close to coming I run images through my head of real and imaginary scenarios such as gangs of filthy tramps all fucking and beating me and then kicking me into the gutter and pissing all over me. I can often have flashes of up to 100 images, real and imagined, before I come. I could go on and on relating them but I think you've got the picture by now. I do not want these things in reality but I have *acted* out lots of them. I do feel I have to be careful who I tell these fantasies to, for obvious reasons.

Sex is very important, but perhaps even more important is my brain. I need it to be filled up. My lovers have to engage my brain to get the best out of me. I only have sex with friends I can trust.

Avedon Carol, a founding member of Feminists Against Censorship, is the author of Nudes, Prudes and Attitudes: Pornography and Censorship *(New Clarion Press, Gloucestershire, 1994) and co-edited* Bad Girls & Dirty Pictures: The Challenge to Reclaim Feminism *(Pluto Press, London & Boulder, 1993). She also serves on the executive committee for the National Council for Civil Liberties ("Liberty"). She has been an activist on civil rights and anti-war issues since she was a teenager in the 1960s and still has the scars to prove it. After moving from the Washington, DC area to London in 1985, she was astonished to find herself in a "free" country where even members of the press and the opposition take for granted that censorship is the best way to solve social problems.*

Body Parts

Avedon Carol

I'm not sure when I started to feel that pornography was an affront to me. Bit by bit, I suppose, I reacted to the sense of exclusion: this was one of any number of things that were supposed to be of interest only to men, and thus evidence that females weren't quite like real people. Of course, the same was true of *Sports Illustrated* and other magazines about sports — or, for that matter, sports themselves — but at least I knew women who were involved with sports, who loved to watch professional football and played basketball, so that wasn't so bad.

But pornography? Who liked pornography? Only guys. And it seemed very strange to me that men seemed to be interested in looking at pictures of complete strangers naked, or movies of strangers having sex with each other. I couldn't imagine that women would want to do that.

I was wrong, of course. I guess the women who did like pornography knew better than to talk to me about it, and maybe they knew better than to hang around with me in the first place.

But the principal reaction I always had to pornography was that it was boring. And sometimes it was downright crass, I thought. I mean, why would people want to look at those disgusting body parts, anyway?

Like a lot of young women, I began to suspect that there was something seriously wrong with men. And it was very easy to think that pornography was some sort of emblem of everything that was wrong with men. The way people always talked about "hardcore", well, I just assumed that this was some sort of pornography that demonstrated just how depraved and repulsive men really were.

Eventually I had to look at a lot of porn for a paper I was working on, and I began to realize that all the terrible things I had come to believe about pornography weren't true. It was still mostly boring, but I couldn't find all the violence and male dominance everyone was always talking about. I suppose that was a bit of a disappointment, really.

But unconsciously, while I was looking at all this porn, it was certainly having an effect on me. It didn't occur to me until well after the paper was written, handed in, graded and returned, but I had just stopped feeling that there was something wrong with my own body.

My relationship with certain body parts had not been very good. I was okay with legs, faces, hair, arms, backs, and even breasts and backsides, most of the time, but when it came to genitals I was not very comfortable. Male genitals were strange and wrinkly and spilled out all over the place like so many triffids. I remember the first time I saw them I thought it was a lucky thing for boys they were located someplace where people wouldn't notice them and they could be covered up all the time.

My own body had been satisfactory for about the first decade of its existence, but then one day there was some sort of rebellion "down there". Things began to stick out, and there was also this unruly hair that seemed to entirely ruin the tidy effect of what had been a nice, smooth little juncture between my legs. I hadn't even had to notice it before, and pretty much didn't, after all, I wasn't supposed to touch it, anyway), but now there seemed to be things calling for attention, things that were darker and wrinkly and strange (although, thankfully, not quite as strange as boy things). And things started to get a bit gooey, too. I wasn't pleased about this at all.

Inevitably, I got old enough that it became impossible to keep other people from noticing these bits from time to time, too. And in the incomprehensible way of males, they seemed particularly interested in these very same embarrassing bits. You just could not seem to keep them from wanting to get involved in these bits, for some reason, which I thought showed remarkably poor taste on their part. It was entirely confusing that males were neither embarrassed about having yucky bits themselves nor averse to looking at, touching, smelling and even *tasting* yucky bits on girls (and sometimes even on other men). But I suppose it seemed typical of boys that they would like something yucky, and of course that they would think having bigger yucky bits was somehow superior to having only small yucky bits.

But I found it absolutely mortifying that you could be with someone you were falling in love with, and of course you would want to impress them with how nice and sweet and cool and clean and smart you were, and they just wanted to go climbing down and investigate the one part of your body that you just wanted to hide. They would always claim that it smelled nice and was pretty and that they liked the feel and taste of it, but you thought, well, they are surely just saying that to be nice, or to try to convince you that they aren't woman-haters — or else, of course, they are really sick perverts.

And then, naturally, they expected you to return the favour. God! Aside from it being disgusting, it was totally intimidating, because I didn't have the faintest clue what to do with the thing and I was much too cool to ask. It would have been so unsophisticated to ask, of course — "Well, how, exactly, should I do this?" I just would have felt like a complete Martian.

It took me years to get used to cocks. Eventually I did learn how to ask questions and it started to be interesting. I even accepted the fact that, deranged though it seemed, men really *were* interested in those strange bits girls had "down there" and weren't just making it up to be nice, and maybe if so many of them felt that way they weren't perverts, either.

Eventually I was working in a clinic where I did gynaecological work, and I saw more women's genitals. That was better, but I spent most of my time doing counseling and didn't see that many, and a lot of them were much cuter and pinker and a lot less unruly than mine.

But looking at pornography finally seemed to have made the difference. There I was giving myself a pelvic exam one day and I didn't feel like I was putting a brave face on it anymore. It just looked normal — I'd seen dozens of "pink shots" of complete strangers who looked at least as unruly as I did, and now it seemed kind of, well, *neat*. It didn't make me uncomfortable at all anymore. I didn't feel like a freak.

And, feeling less embarrassed about my own body, I felt a lot less embarrassed about letting anyone else see, touch, and even taste it. And I felt a whole new level of curiosity about *their* bodies. Sex with someone else seemed a lot more like a joyous adventure.

When I hear other women complain about pornography, one of the big complaints they make is about those "pink shots". There is one anti-porn campaigner who constantly refers with disgust to what she calls "splayed vaginas". It's as if it's understood: there could be nothing more revolting than to look at cunts. God knows it's hard enough to find them anywhere else — what other genre (other than medical texts -yuck!) shows you women's genitals? Where else do you see them? Only in porn, because porn is the only place where they aren't considered too disgusting to look at.

It says a lot about society when even women who claim to be advocates for women can't stand the sight of pussy and think no one else should want to look at it, either. I felt that way for too long, and I'm glad pornography helped me get over it. Maybe, rather than trying to hide porn, and hide from porn, those women should be spending a whole lot more time looking at it for what it really is — just pictures of the sex and very nice parts of our bodies that our crummy old sexist society wants us to hide and feel ashamed of.

No more of that for me, thanks. I have come to the conclusion that pussy — cunt, quim, whatever — is the best thing that ever happens to most people.

One time Labour party activist and CND supporter; current and very active FAC member and producer of stylish smut, Lesley Sharrock has been writing professionally for eight years. In 1994, she co-founded an erotic magazine with her partner Ian Jackson and sees adult material aimed at both sexes as the way forward for modern erotica.

Adopted child, ex-hippy, mother and soon-to-be-anytime-now grand-mother, Sharrock is also currently researching a book about adopted people as adults and their shared experiences.

PORNUTOPIA

Lesley Ann Sharrock

My first real experience of pornography was in the early 70s when my ex-husband and I were running a newsagents shop in Liverpool. The 'top shelf' didn't exist yet and the softcore market was in its infancy. These were men's magazines and were merely racked-up with everything else. Nobody I encountered was in the least bit offended by this stuff, perhaps because no-body had yet told them that they should be. But apart from the legal fare we also sold under-the-counter hardcore magazines from Germany, which I found to be the real turn-on. The men's mags at that time were full of naked girls; they did not do a lot for me, a dyed-in-the-wool hetero. But within the glossy pages of the iffy stuff were great and not-so-great looking guys with big stiff dicks penetrating every available female orifice. Now that really got the juices flowing! So much so that I would often sneak off to our flat above the shop in the afternoons and mas-turbate using the images as stimulation. This was my unliberated period and I didn't even think to share these experiences with my husband. He'd have thought I was some kind of slut for en-joying it anyway. To his Neanderthal mind, 'nice' women didn't do that sort of thing.

Later, in the mid-eighties, I was divorced, trying to pay an exorbitant mortgage and involved in a relationship of true equals. My partner suggested I try writing for a porn mag to make a few extra pennies and, bugger me, I found that I was pretty good at it. Words I had rarely even spoken flowed from my typewriter like so much sexual lubrication, freeing my formerly conventional mind in a way I had never thought possible. Not only did I become comfortable with the word cunt but with the reality of my own. I realised what a sheltered life I had been living, how repressed by the pedestal and how honest I was now able to be about my own sexuality. This was almost a Road To Damascus experience for me. A discovery on a par with that of Tutankhamen's tomb!

Not an intellectual exercise by any stretch of the imagination, I wrote explicit crudery full of dripping this and throbbing that. Pricks, cunts, cocks and arses quivered and writhed with abandon within my lubricious prose. Not for me the rising manhood or lubricating vagina, oh dear me, no. The heavier and juicier it got the better I liked it. My imagination reined-in only by the constraints of the law and the publishers' fear of prosecution. Obscene publications be damned, I thought, get a load of this!

The more I wrote, and sold, the prouder I became of my minor achievement. And, innocent that I was, when asked what I did I'd say so loud and clear. Then one day I was shocked. Not by something I had written but by people's reaction to it; the horrified looks from friends I had previously thought of as being liberal and free-thinking; the general distaste of some or the lecherous innuendo from some friends' husbands who thought that my new-found notoriety meant I was easy meat. With friends like that, I thought, who needs enemas! So, instead of either hiding or changing my occupation, I changed my friends.

From a pin-money hobby pornography has become a full-time occupation. In fact, my partner and I have founded our own company to produce *Desire*, the first British erotic magazine for couples. For, while I wildly applaud all the new erotica for women, I feel the next step has to be to bring the sexes together. Ex-husbands apart, I feel the similarities between the sexes are greater than the differences. This has become all the more obvious to me because we use both male and female writers and photographers in *Desire* and I defy anyone to be able to tell from much of the work submitted whether a man or a woman has produced it.

I also believe that the more honest we can be with each other about our sexual needs, wants and cravings, the closer we can become. It has certainly worked for me in my present relationship. And it seems to me that those who wish to protect the status quo of separation of the sexes are desperately trying to shift their own fears of human sexuality onto the rest of us.

Since having such intimate involvement with the genre, for that is what it is, I have come to realise a few things. For example, porn is often criticised for being fantasy-based but you have to ask why should pornography be realistic? Nobody condemns crime stories, romantic fiction or the Western for being products of the imagination, so why should porn be any different?

Also, I have often thought of pornography in the terms of any expressive medium: cinema, art, books, etc. What is it that people find offensive and why? Why is the high body count of an Arnie shoot-em-up movie okay yet *Reservoir Dogs* and *Natural Born Killers* get stomped on? Well nobody is going to become emotionally caught up with 'Terminator 12' are they, because it's really just Tom and Jerry meets Mighty Mouse. And, historically, the more uninvolving or abstract the work the less likely it is to be censored. But viewing the horrifically realistic blood-letting of *Reservoir Dogs* involves the feelings whether they be excitement or revulsion. So as any work moves further away from ideas or caricature and into the realms of the emotional senses the hackles of the repressed begin to rise.

Pornography aims to arouse, something many people are uncomfortable with. And it works. Most people are aroused — whether they admit it or not — by porn, thereby evoking strong emotions. The words used by the anti-porn lobby, 'demeaning', 'obscene', 'offensive', 'immoral' are, to my mind, merely a smokescreen for their own personal discomfort with explicit imagery. But, let's face it, nobody has the God-given right to go through life without being offended or caused discomfort. And anyway, these things are a learning experience and can often be good for you. And they extend throughout our lives.

During an illness which the family was convinced would bump her off, my eighty-six year old grandmother got hooked on Saturday-afternoon televised wrestling matches. She watched with wide, rheumy-eyed, gob-smacked fascination as some snarling and sweaty 'baddie' crashed the good guy against the ropes then used him as a human trampoline. 'It shouldn't be allowed!' I can still hear her cry. But she watched every week, rooted to her chair and loving every moment. Finding this new interest, she survived another four years, her vocabulary liberally peppered with such terms as, 'arm lock', 'full Nelson' and, her particular favourite, 'back slam'. That was the 1960s, but had she still been around, she'd have been glued to the far sexier Gladiators.

As a preteen visiting a fairground with friends, I can remember shaking with trepidation as I approached The Ghost Train, The Big Dipper or The Waltzers. I was terrified and exhilarated all at once. And, after practically wetting myself, I went back for more.

My first sexual experience brought out similar conflicting emotions. I was fourteen years old and a classmate and I would sneak off to his house at lunchtime when his mother was at work to 'do it'. The most amusing thing that happened was when, after one of our grope-and-poke sessions we got back to school to be confronted by a red-faced male teacher who informed the class that we were about to have sex education. John, my partner in guilt-laden pleasures, passed me a note which read 'what does he want to know?' But, looking back, just how little we knew was bloody frightening. Sex education was too little and too late. We knew nothing about contraception and it was just pure blind luck that I didn't become a teenage pregnancy statistic. And, abortion being illegal at that time, been driven into a marriage that would have been far more disastrous than the one I entered into of my own free will.

Sexual repression touches us all, whether it is lack of sex education, inability to communicate with sexual partners or general ignorance of the possibilities for sexual fulfillment that explicit material can present. I, for one, can say that pornography changed my life, my way of thinking and my ability to admit — even to myself— the boundaries of my sexual existence. And I will fight to my last breath the repression of sexual expression that is so much a part of our society. Straight or gay, we are all in this struggle together and should slug it out shoulder to shoulder for a better and more sexually tolerant world.

By the way, my ex-husband is still very uncomfortable with what I do for a living. Although the daughter of our loins thinks it's great! One up to me, I think.

After training at Art College, both fine art and history of, Caroline Bottomley took a job designing posters at the Leadmill, a nightclub, venue and arts centre in Sheffield, England. She enjoyed it so much she stayed and did, amongst other things: promoting 'the best small scale arts season in the country', (with drunken performance artists and theatre directors who wanted directions to the best brothels after the show); managing major new building projects — and mucking in with demolishing a toilet block . . . never again; and finally running the commercial programme of the Leadmill with over 400 gigs and club nights a year. Bottomley's got an MBA and Marketing Diploma, studied for whilst at the Leadmill, and now she's starting her own sex toy business.

NO NO YES

Caroline Bottomley

I've got two stories about buying vibrators. The first one is about when I went to an Ann Summers party. If you haven't ever been to one, the principle is that women get their women friends and a small truckload of alcohol round to someone's house, where a rep gently leads you through a progression of the various goods on offer, speed is dictated by the amount of alcohol and drinking capacity of those concerned.

So, we all began to get drunk and we all giggled a lot playing "pin the penis on the man" warm-up games and looking at saucy playing cards. Then we got to lingerie, and I was the one chosen to go and put on the PVC playsuit. I appeared to the sound of the front room humming like the Tardis; this is what we were waiting for — the rep had got out the hard stuff.

Everybody had a vibrator in their hands — and what was happening? Everyone was holding them against cheeks and backs and saying oh yes, what good body massagers they are, really good for when you've got stiff neck. Giggle giggle we all went. And at the end of the party and despite being well plastered, we went into a slightly embarrassed silence while we furtively filled out our order forms.

I decided to pick the rudest looking vibrator on offer as an act of bravado, but felt a bit nervous about being the odd one out. It had the lot; a wiggly squirming action, multi speed vibrations and various appendages for reaching the parts that other vibrators just wouldn't reach.

Group approval had definitely been for the small, cream colored, inoffensive six incher. I found out later from the rep that was what most people had ordered. No one really wanted to let on about what they'd bought — very few women owned up to buying one of the vibrators. Certainly none of us swapped notes after the party about whether their vibrator was any good or not (mine was lots of fun by the way). We'd had fun, we'd had a laugh, and we all felt as though we'd done something naughty.

So sex is fun, and a laugh; and passionate, and serious. And there's all sorts of special frissons about feeling you're doing something forbidden, or something very private. But it seems to me there are other limiting and constricting censorious voices at play here. Saying 'you're not supposed to' and 'nice girls don't'.

Despite the image women like to have of women, I think they're still very much at work. Owning up to using sex toys is taboo — it's ok to buy products that improve your health, or alter your appearance, but not to buy ones that are solely about sexual pleasure. And I've observed that holds true for a lot of men too.

Despite the fact that men are by far and away the biggest purchasers of sex toys, a common public response in discussions about vibrators and so on is that they feel quite threatened by them. There's a definite interest in them in general. When you get down to personal specifics, attitudes gravitate toward perfomance, 'I don't need that sort of thing'.

The roles of naughty children and stern parents seem to typify much of the public attitude to sex in this country, which of course has an impact on everyone's private beliefs. But there is change, there is a lot more discussion about sex going on in the public arena. Are we moving toward more adult attitudes toward sex? There's certainly a significant amount of people that are trying to shape attitudes that way. A lot of them are women, and I think that's no coincidence. Saying what you think, saying what you feel, women are famous for 'being in touch with our emotions'. So it's not surprising that there are more honest and more diverse discussions about sex and sexuality as more women consider and promote what they think and feel about sex.

Pornography, (definition; "the writing of harlots") and media debates — "the writing of (fill in your own words depending on which media you're thinking of)" are both notably developing different flavors and trends, albeit in a small but still significant way. Enough people feel confident enough to be brave and honest about how they really feel about powerful subjects like sex, and a lot of those people are women.

The Ann Summers story happened 15 years ago. My other story is happening now. I'm buying vibrators in bulk. Not because I'm consumed with a mad desire for constant mechanical stimulation in all forms imaginable, but because I'm starting to sell them by mail order.

I like using vibrators, they do a good job, and a wham pow whew orgasm brightens up anyone's day. I think there's a gap in the marketplace for well presented, stylish products. I guess there's a lot of people out there, men and women, who don't want to feel like they're wandering down streets of slime by purchasing sex products.

Of course your mental attitude to something is within your control — you can make your own judgments about whether what you're doing is seedy or not. But its also formed by what's around you, and there's times when I've felt quite heartsick researching this business, let me tell you why. I found out who the main and mysterious suppliers are in this country, then began the task of poring over their catalogues; what looks good, what looks like it would really be pleasurable to use, what seems down-right daft (a vibrator that not only vibrates but moans to you while you're using it? hmmm), and what seems like a con (have you ever heard anyone say that penis enlarger cream really has given them a bigger dick?).

So far so good. Ok, so I don't like the look of the catalogues, but that's why I think theres a place for a new approach. But after a while, I began to feel sick of seeing women posed in "dying for it" positions, with brain dead expressions on their faces. Irritated, subjugated, subdued, tainted. Cross. And that's the effect a lot of 'pornography' has on me after a while. It's not because I'm looking at pictures about sex, what offends me is all the other messages in there about 'what women are like,' 'what women are for'.

On the subject of another form of pornography, how many sex videos have I seen with attractive women being passive and paunchy men, yes usually with socks on, pumping away monotonously in the grim aim of getting to the cum shots. Reminds me of watching hamsters running on wheels. Whenever I've been watching with female friends, it invariably ends up with us ranting on about how downright crap the videos are. We're not turned on, we're belligerent. There's obviously something of value in there and maybe there is something a bit sexy about seeing people having sex — it wouldn't be the huge industry it is otherwise. But I feel at odds with the idea that this is what I can buy into as 'sexy', when it has so little soul.

I feel in danger of getting censorious now about what is 'good' sex and what is 'bad'. Thats not the point — I think most pornography is crap, unimaginative and uncreative. It can be responded to fearfully, because often it's got aggressive messages about women in it. No viewpoint, no voice from the women involved or the women who might be watching or reading it. I mean, there I go, suspending my disbelief in order to get into a story, a book or a video, and I think no way! If I was there I'd want to get up and cover his bum in baby oil, or swap dirty stories with him, or try it on top of the washing machine, or play at harems with fifteen other people, or dungeons, or foreign prisons on exotic islands (I digress) or almost anything at all. But merely pouting and looking available doesn't do a lot for me, doesn't really fit with my idea of my place in the world and who I want to be.

There is pornography out there which turns me on, and I know that there's more coming all the time. Good for Candida Royalle's videos — which aren't actually that good 'cause we're in Britain and the censor's taken all the fun bits out. Good for Annie Sprinkle, and I wish I could buy your videos over here as well. Good for Tuppy Owens and her Sex Maniac activities. Good for Tim Woodward, who's made an interest in S/M & fetishism a more publicly legitimate activity with *Skin 2*, good for all the other thousands of harlots who send out public messages about fun, exciting, scary, passionate,loving, hedonistic, strange, quiet, noisy sex where everybody can enjoy it, and take part in it, and explore their own desires. From my point of view, I've yet to find whether theres a big enough demand out there from people who are fed up of being spoken to as though they're sleaze balls when they're buying sex toys. Perhaps people like things just the way they are, if you don't, look out for me. The company's called NoNoYes!

Marisa Carr is the other half of Dragon Ladies — a feminist based performance company founded with Cherie Matrix. In October 1994, Carr organized, curated and produced a vaudevillian revue of international queer performing artists and dancers exploring issues of sexual politics. With the sponsorship of Feminists Against Censorship and the Leydig Trust, she brought a Smutfest *to Britain.*

Carr has been performing, producing, and devising theatre/live art for four years. She has developed a unique style and approach to performance concerning sexual politics that has been shown in a hugely diverse range of venues and events, from seasons at the ICA in London to Underground Clubs in New York, the Brighton Festival (England) and gay and women's events in Britain and Europe.

I Would . . .

Marisa Carr

When I was a little girl I would sit on the arm of the sofa right at the end. I would push down hard against my jeans so that my knickers would ride up between my legs. I remember this sensation to be especially rewarding when by accident I got to see something sexual on the TV.

I can remember the three main sexual fantasies I had as a girl and I'm sure these were all partly inspired by various films or TV programmes. It may be debatable as to whether these were 'sexual fantasies' or a confused adolescent imagination inwhich sex played a major role.

If by chance my mother was out for the evening, which was very rare, my father would let me stay up much later, and it was on one of these occasions I chanced to see a scene from *Oh Lucky Man*, a film with Malcolm Macdowell. (I only realised it was a scene in this film when I saw it again as a young woman.)

Now, in this film, the main character goes to a men's club, where hostesses sit on the laps of businessmen and strippers perform shows on a stage. This gave me a fascination with sex shows that I still have to this very day. I think what turned me on is the idea of people watching the woman and in my fantasies I would be both the business man and the stripper.

I was always very fond of anything to do with the 'Orient', my particular favourites being Peter Sellers as 'Fu Man Chu' and Bruce Lee in *Enter the Dragon*. Both involved Mafioso secret societies housed in exotic hideaways inhabited by well toned kung fu fighters and harems of voluptuous silk clad hostesses. In my fantasy I was one of a number of female captives in a labyrinth of caves being led on a chain, semi-naked and dirty (in a ripped leather slave girl outfit reminiscent of Raquel Welch in *2,000,000 BC*) to the 'Emperor' who was to decide our terrible fate.

He was on a high ornate throne with a long black moustache and in front of him was a deep green pool of water, which was full of man eating piranhas. We were pushed into a human sized gold bird cage and suspended twenty feet above the pool, squashed up against each other's breasts and thighs. We clung naked together as the floor of the cage started to give way.

The colours of my fantasies were Technicolor like *Enter the Dragon* or the *Wizard of Oz*, or like a Roger Corman horror movie — like Vincent Price in *The Pit and the Pendulum*, which brings me to my final fantasy. This was definitely the most frightening and was a mixture of sex and horror.

I used to imagine that there was a man in my wardrobe who had black hair, deadly white skin, long fingernails and red eyes. (This image was very much connected with Ziggy Stardust.) He cane out of my closet and did sexual things with me. I was frightened and *not* frightened by him, he was charming and horrific at the same time.

Years later, when talking to friends about whether we masturbated as girls, I couldn't remember that I ever had — because I don't recall outrightly taking my hand to my vagina and doing it with that intention in mind.

We also talked about porn. Do women really 'get off' on images the men do? For me, my earliest experiences of masturbation are inextricably linked with bits of films of people in sexually evocative situations.

Wholly unconscious of the fact that I was masturbating and 'getting off' on the images, I was quite addicted to conjuring them up in my mind, whilst pushing up and down against the family furniture.

Carol Leigh is an artist, feminist, hooker, activist and video maker who lives in San Francisco. Her first play, in which she played herself, back in 1982, was the first performance about the stigma of sex work; in fact, she invented the name "Sex Worker". Her nick-name The Scarlet Harlot comes from her red hair and wild appearance. Carol is hoping to develop her genre of esoteric sex education videos and become a Great Pornographer.

The Scarlet Harlot

Carol Leigh

My father had a pornography collection which my mother insisted he hide in the cupboard under the stairs. Since I knew where it was, whenever they went out of the house, to go shopping or whatever, I got a chair so I could reach up and get out the magazines.

One of the magazines had a beautiful woman in it. Her name was Carol, just like mine, and she was posed under a Christmas tree, looking so friendly, and so beautiful and loving. I wanted to grow up and be just like her, with my breasts pert and everything. So, that's what I imagined I would be, although I repressed that desire a lot.

My mother resented the pornography collection because she thought it gave my father some extra power. She felt the porn was an insult to her. Dad was nasty to her — he didn't work much, he was lazy, and not really that accommodating. I loved my mother, who was lovely and beautiful and kind. My father was twenty eight when they married and my mother only seventeen. She was a virgin when they met and he wasn't. He was more aggressive sexually and, although they did have a hot relationship, she said she felt like a prostitute sometimes, because he'd pressure her. So there was a discourse in my family all the time.

My parents strongly believed that people should be able to talk openly about sexuality, so they discussed it and were naked in front of us (although not sexual) until we were twelve or so. There was a freedom which went both ways: I became free and open but I was aware of the imbalance of power. I could observe him chasing her, being verbally abusive. So, sexuality meant a combination of those two things.

My parents thought they should teach me about sex, but sadly, it was my father who taught me, from text book, when I was in bed. This felt awkward and wrong. I wished my mother had done it. My sexual history was confusing. I started getting involved with boys when I was fifteen or sixteen. I had guilt mixed up with lots of issues, so I'd go only so far with boys, then stop. I realised I could hardly get aroused: as soon as we started doing it, I wasn't aroused at all. I was afraid I was frigid even though I was pretty open minded.

I realised that I was bisexual from a very early age, after a big relationship with a girl when I was nine. Thus, I knew I didn't want to be monogamous. I became a feminist when I was twenty one. I started going to lesbian bars, and met lesbian feminists. I started masquerading as a lesbian while refusing to admit I was bisexual. I was still trying to work it out with men.

I was sort of anti-porn at that point. As a feminist, I was supposed to come out about the different ways I appeared as a woman, which meant lying about my sexuality. The way women spoke about men was incredibly insulting to them. I didn't mind sharing my problems, but didn't like insulting men *en masse*. It was very difficult for me, confusing. I was fantasizing about doing sex work, and playing out these fantasies with my boyfriend. But as a feminist, I knew I shouldn't be doing that.

One of my closest friends, Macha Womongold, was the anti-porn activist who shot a bullet through a window of a shop selling sex magazines in Harvard Square in Boston, and had her children taken away as a result. She switched to environmentalism after that. She'd been the one to bring me into feminism, taught me about the Goddess, even though she was dating a stripper. I had met her at Graduate School, where I had gone to study with Ann Sexton.

My sex life took on the image I had of my Mum — I assumed that she was offended by my dad, his verbal abuse and his porno collection but, in actual, fact my Mum was aroused by all this in an S/M kind of way and it kept her addicted to the relationship.

I moved to San Francisco after school, when Ann Sexton had killed herself. I was on the verge of breaking up with a boyfriend, and needed money. I saw ads for sex massage girls. I thought I was desperate, so why don't I just go there and do it? I went to the sleaziest parlour, to make sure I picked one that wasn't selling anything else, like glamour! Once I started work, I was enchanted by the women, to see how they deal with their roles. I met women from all around the world, from Vietnam, Korea, Mexico, and I'd never had the chance to be with sexually wise, strong women before — it was really exciting. The men would come in, pay you, come and, before you know it, it was over! Then you have all this money! As soon as I tried it, I knew it was going to be my life's work.

I was already a committed artist, almost twenty eight and looking for something to write about. I remembered Gloria Steinem who infiltrated *Playboy* and became a bunny and trashed them, and I thought, well if she can trash *Playboy*, I should investigate prostitution.

T. Grace Atkinson said that prostitutes are in the front way in the battle of the sexes. I'd studied Hemingway, and Hemingway went to war to write about it. I decided to do the same with prostitution. I was fascinated. I looked in the mirror and said "Oh. that's a prostitute." I'd always heard that you couldn't turn back after you'd stepped over that line from the good girl to the bad. That was a dare for me. How could it be that I could never turn back after one hand job? I remember feeling, after I'd crossed the line, that I turned round, and the line had disappeared. Imagine walking into your whole life's work. It made sense. After all, I was doing prostitution with my boyfriends, now I was getting paid for it. It all fitted together. The more I did it, the more I learned about sex, and the less scary sex became. It wasn't a cure-all, although I've had the best sex in my personal life when I've been working most, because the work inspired me sexually. I had a lover at the beginning and my relationship with him was very erotic. What I enjoyed about the work was the way I didn't really like it with my tricks, and how this contrasted with the way they thought I did like it with them. On the other hand, if I had a few things that were quasi arousing during the day, I'd have a good time with my boyfriend that night.

When I first started working as a prostitute, I went along to a meeting of the National Organisation for Women, with a paper bag on my head, on which was written "This paper bag symbolizes the anonymity prostitutes are forced to adopt." I realised that I had a role as a feminist.

The title of my play, "The Adventures of Scarlet Harlot, the Demystification of the Sex Work Industry", was sort of a joke, but I knew we needed a word that was different than prostitute. Now the expression "Sex Worker" is used around the world, and it's changed the movement and people's concepts. I'm really proud of that. It's brought the strippers and peep show workers and prostitutes together. I had studied linguistics at college and, after all that training, it was great to be able to put it to some use!

The play used my poetry, and I'd wander into the audience and ask them what they did for a living and sneer, saying they were whores too. It was a fun piece and I had loads of press. I took lessons in acting and singing. My play was about stigma but, when the AIDS crisis came along, suddenly the issue wasn't stigma so much any more, the issue was AIDS. I was totally traumatized because, at the beginning, there was no way to get tested. Every day, I heard more about prostitutes spreading this terrible disease and the tricks refused to use condoms.

So I decided I'd leave San Francisco and become a Country and Western star in Austin, Texas. I was going to form an organisation, Texas Whores and Tricks — TWAT! Fortunately, my car broke down in Tucson, where they had all these strip joints I reckoned I could work in. This was where I met Dave Bukunus, an artist and video maker, through an ad in a paper. He worked at TWIT, Tucson Western International Television, so I set out to do TWAT but ended up doing TWIT. We had a great affair and he taught me everything about making video. I wrote, directed and edited public access comedy videos.

Eventually, I returned to San Francisco and started working with Citizens for Medical Justice, the organisation which preceded ACT-UP. I was a founder member of the Cal-Act and joined the Sisters of Perpetual Indulgence. We staged demonstrations against the church and censorship, and I did a lot of political art and activist work. Nowadays, I'm city government, I'm the main organizer of the City Task Force on Prostitution, and we are winning — we're in the process of decriminalizing prostitution in San Francisco but it's definitely a long project. We want the whores to be in charge, not the management! Prostitution works best as a cottage industry. Our main goal is an on-going panel with a majority of sex workers on it, to monitor working conditions, police, etc.

I still work as a whore but only with regular clients. Not many activists still work full time although some do. Dolores French is still dedicated to the work itself. I still do outreach work with street prostitutes. A lot of the discussion is around street prostitutes, they are symbols of the poverty today.

The first sex video I was involved in was Annie Sprinkle's *Sluts and Goddesses* video. Annie is fabulous and lovely and generous and professional. It was really hot in the studio in New York, we were very sweaty, so it was hard. Being in New York was handy because it meant I was near my father, who was dying on Long Island. He died the day after the shoot finished.

My own personal fantasies are submissive and so the pornography I like to view personally shows women being tied up.

I need to be forced because I feel very guilty but that's only in game-playing, and I know the difference. I enjoy watching one woman being screwed by a group of men, with lots of penises everywhere.

Since 1985, I have been recording the cultural underground in terms of sexual rights and now my videos are more pornographic. Esoteric sex education is what I call my style of work, but I need a better name. I feel my genre has a long way to go, although I'm glad that people want the Scarlet Harlot touch.

Joe Kramer, Annie Sprinkle, Dorrie Lane all work in this new genre, and I help interpret their ideas, by being their director and editor of their films. I'm helping them express their vision. What I really want to make is a sex comedy. Somebody gave me a cute title: "Genitals — the Comedy," and I want to make it! — porn which crosses over the markets. I'm more comfortable mocking sex than exploring the rhythms of lust. I like sexual imagery that is funny. I want to be a great pornographer. Amongst the greatest — with Henry Miller. Andrea Dworkin is a great pornographer. Annie Sprinkle is a great pornographer and her *Sluts And Goddesses* video is one of the best pornographic videos. Kay Diamond's ejaculation video was great too. But if there's great erotic comedy to be made now, I would like to make it. I see that as my future. The Monty Python of Sex.

Carol Queen is a writer and sex educator who specializes in articulating the experience and issues of marginalized sexualities. She is about to get her doctorate in sexology with an emphasis on erotic literature, and directs the continuing education program for the workers at Good Vibrations, San Francisco's "friendly, feminist and fun" sex toy shop. Her erotic writing and essays have appeared in Best American Erotica, Heretica, The Erotic Impulse, Doing It for Daddy, Madonnarama, Women of the Light, Cafe Sex, *and many other anthologies. Her first book,* Exhibitionism for the Shy, *is available from Down There Press; her second, co-edited with Lawrence Schimel and published by Cleis, is* Switch Hitters: Lesbians Write Gay Male Erotica and Gay Men Write Lesbian Erotica. *She lives in San Francisco, yet is constantly travelling.*

The Four Foot Phallus

Carol Queen

I was an anti-pornography feminist. Everything the anti-porn feminists said made perfect sense to me. Those movies were just awful. No prude, I. I had a very grandiose way of explaining my opposition to pornography. It wasn't that the movies were dirty and explicit, no. "Pornography," I would sigh, as if the topic was slightly boring but also hurt me personally, "always insults either my intelligence, my political sensibilities, or my sense of the erotic." Nobody ever said, "How many movies have you seen?" I had seen precisely two x-rated movies in my life, plus read a handful of *Penthouse Letters.* (Actually, I didn't mind the letters, though the dirty words were as embarrassing as they were titillating.)

This state of affairs persisted until I went away to graduate school in sexology. At my school they meant us to watch porn. They wanted us, they said, to become "desensitized" to it. For the first week they showed rather tame things, explicit movies made for sex education. All very nice. But then it was time for the desensitization part. The instructors said they had something very special to show us, and put out the lights. We were in a large room with high-ceilinged white walls. Suddenly patch after patch of the white wall lit up with color and motion. "The Fuckarama!" the instructor announced proudly. "You're seeing seventeen different images!"

Each patch was a different movie. One was an old circa 1970 heterosexual fuck scene. The woman had a truly ridiculous hairdo and the man had the most outrageous sideburns I'd seen since, well, 1970. But they were having what looked like a rollicking fuck. Another screen held two men in a restroom. Now *this* was interesting. But what were they doing *pissing* on each other?

Then a transsexual one started up. The woman in it had a penis. Fetish. S/M. Lesbian three-ways. Interracial scenes. A woman with a dog. Grainy, scratchy black and white porn from the 30s, the 40s, the 50s. Elephants fucking! Everything was up on the wall! One scene after another caught my eye. I was surrounded by larger-than-life fucking, sucking, fisting— a Great Wall of Sex. However, the promised desensitization didn't seem to be happening to me; my clit was positively buzzing. Everything made me horny, even things I'd never seen before, even things I thought I'd never do.

I was desperately thankful the lights were out. I began to watch one scene closely, at first not understanding what I found so compelling about it. It was just a heterosexual cocksucking scene, nothing very special. Except that it was shot very, very close-up. The woman's lips were huge. You could only see from her mouth to the fringe of her eyelashes. And the man's cock must have taken up four feet of wall. I don't remember if it struck me right then, or if the awareness came bubbling up from a part of me that wasn't conscious of the thought process — but when the lights were back on and the instructors asked us to tell them how watching the Fuckarama had felt, I raised my hand and blurted out, "I realized while watching this that I had never actually *looked* at a penis before!" They nodded at me gravely. They were used to all sorts of revelations from first-time viewers of the Fuckarama.

Their response was anti-climactic; looking back, I realize that was one of the top five most important moments I've ever had, sexually speaking. To understand, first, that I really had no idea what porn was all about — in the space of forty minutes I saw twenty times as many pornographic images as I'd seen in my whole life — and then to realize that I'd avoided looking at a cock, even though I'd been just as close to plenty of them as the woman in the fellatio movie: it could only mean I was on some level afraid of cocks, and understanding that I had constructed my sexual belief system to cover up my own weak points was a profoundly important realization. It meant I could begin to move away from the place I'd been stuck for so many years.

I became a porno monster. Freed from the "porn is degrading to women" rubric (how easy it was now to understand why I'd embraced that way of viewing it!), I just wanted to watch all I could. I was a sexologist-in-training, of course, so it was all relevant to my studies. But I watched it with my hands deep in my pants, masturbating like there was no tomorrow. It was as if I'd never masturbated before — though, I assure you, I had, and plenty — because the moving images on the screen engaged me erotically like nothing else ever had. I was put into a delicious trance, focused on a cock pumping out of a pussy or an asshole — I didn't care what genders and acts I was viewing, because now the pornography seemed like a wonderland of tumescent, flushing, gasping lust, caught on film just for me.

I volunteered to catalogue porn movies for the school. I took five or six videos home every night. I didn't have a lover and for once didn't even miss it — I was getting more sex than I ever had, from my own hand — and with the full participation of the sexual athletes who crowded the videos, putting on outrageous shows just for me.

When one is as sexually charged as I was, one doesn't go without a lover for very long, I suppose. I met and got involved with an extraordinary man (whose penis I have never been frightened to look at!), and he turned out to be a porn aficionado too, though not a born-again one, as I was. Still, he was just as evangelical in his zeal for dirty movies (in fact, he's in the bedroom as I write this, watching porn). I reached new heights of pleasure when we watched them together, making love or — wonderful discovery! — masturbating right next to each other, breathlessly commenting on the movie while we wanked.

What is it about pornography? I don't think I could have told you then what it was about it that got me so hot. Now that I'm a trained sexologist, I can venture a few interpretations. Who among us is allowed to be as voyeuristic as we might wish to be? Most of us are curious about other people's sexuality, and porn lets us indulge that curiosity with a frank stare (in fact, with a rewind control!). I love porn because, very simply, it lets me watch. Some porn also includes erotic talk and the rich auditory overlay of fucking: gasps, grunts, dirty words whispered or shouted, bodies slapping wetly together. Even if you're still a bit frightened of or offput by the visuals, close your eyes and listen to a porn vid sometime. It's sexual symphony. (Of course, some pornos just feature that execrable muzak.)

Sex therapists often tell people having trouble orgasming to find a method to get out of their heads — stop thinking about whether orgasm will come, whether you're doing it right, and focus on the sensation. That always struck me as advice rather like the direction given to novice meditators: empty your head of all thoughts. Very easy to say, yet hard to do! With the right porn video on, though, you can count on sexy distraction from the voices inside your head — I always find that orgasm sneaks up on me and feels more intense when I have the visuals of a porn movie to simultaneously inspire and distract me.

Plus watching porn is educational in its own right. Never take its actors for templates of eroticism; don't think you ought to be assuming those exact same positions (some of them were only developed for the camera angles they allow!); but how often, as I said before, do we really get to watch? It's fascinating to see what people really do, and I always find things in porn I think I might like to do, too. Whether or not I ever actually try them, they feed my fantasy life — an important aspect of sexuality in its own right.

When I watch with a partner, porn fills yet another function. We can point out to each other erotic aspects, get ideas for frisky erotic experimentation, use it to inspire conversations in which we share preferences, fantasies, history. Porn helps break the ice of erotic conversation.

Once you've gotten comfortable with porn, maybe you'll begin to wonder what it would be like to star in a porn video. Thanks to easily available video cameras, you can! You needn't see them sold in the neighborhood porn shop; you can keep them at home to enjoy. My first turns in front of the camera were silly yet intensely erotic — it was sexy to be filmed, and seeing myself played back on the monitor changed my self-image — I realized how erotic I am when my gaze was uninterrupted by the self-talk that usually accompanies looking at myself in the mirror.

Never mind that I don't look like the frighteningly aerobicized bodies I see in contemporary porn. What I expect from a porno movie is sexual energy, seeing sex embodied in a person or people — whom I can voyeuristically enjoy; when that person is myself, it's a powerful experience — much more powerful than I ever expected. Besides, stepping in front of the camera lets me revel in my exhibitionism — even if no one but me and my lover will ever see the results.

I owe a lot to that four-foot phallus — a much deeper acquaintance with my own eroticism, for starters. And it's such a wonderful change not to feel afraid of sex any more. Finally, it lets me look at the world very differently, thinking that sexual entertainment is for me, too — not just for men. That is every bit as feminist as the ill-thought-through (and frightfully inexperienced) beliefs I started out with about porn.

Feminists Against Censorship

Feminists Against Censorship (FAC) was formed in London, England in 1989 to give a voice to the many anti-censorship feminists who felt they were being silenced by the anti-pornography movement, which purported to represent a desire on the part of all women, and all feminists, to censor pornography. At the time the group was founded, there was virtually no debate on censorship in the UK. We believe we have made a difference.

We have been described as both a "campaigning group" and a "pressure group", but to a large extent we see our role as educational, both in terms of making people aware of the long anti-censorship history in feminism and the varying attitudes women hold, and clarifying what the research really shows about media, violence, and social attitudes. We hope our books serve as a means to help people find this information more easily.

Obviously, given our initial brief, only women can make policy and speak for FAC, but we are not separatist and welcome people of all sexes and sexualities to become supporters, receive our newsletters, and come to our public events.

Similar groups have been formed in North America, beginning with FACT, the Feminist Anti-Censorship Taskforce. In the 1990s, Feminists for Free Expression (FFE) was formed in New York and has been campaigning actively ever since.

CONTACT INFO:

Feminists Against Censorship
BM Box 207
London WC1N 3XX
ENGLAND
Phone: (0181) 552-4405
avedon@cix.compulink.co.uk
http://www.fullfeed.com/hypatia/
censor.html

In the US, contact:

Feminists for Free Expression
2525 Times Square Station
New York, NY 10108
FFE@aol.com
http://www.well.com/user/freedom

National Coalition Against Censorship
275 7th Avenue
New York, NY 10001
NCAC@netcom.com

New from AK Press

SCUM Manifesto by Valerie Solanas. ISBN 1-873176 44-9; 64 pp, two color cover, perfect bound 5-1/2 x 8-1/2; £3.50/$5.00. This is the definitive edition of the SCUM Manifesto with an afterword detailing the life and death of Valerie Solanas. "Life in this society being, at best, an utter bore and no aspect of society being at all relevant to women, there remains to civic-minded, responsible, thrill-seeking females only to overthrow the government, eliminate the money system, institute complete automation and destroy the male sex. . . . On the shooting of Andy

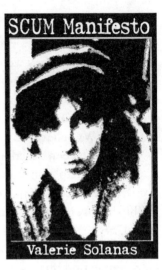

Warhol: I consider that a moral act. And I consider it immoral that I missed. I should have done target practice." —Valerie Solanas

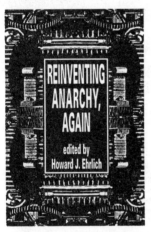

Reinventing Anarchy, Again edited by Howard J. Ehrlich. ISBN 1-873176 88-0; 400pp, two color cover, perfect bound 6x9; £13.95/$19.95. A fully revised and updated printing of this seminal work of contemporary anarchism, theory and practice, the first edition of which sold over 20,000 copies. Reinventing Anarchy, Again brings together the major currents of social anarchist theory in a collection of some of the most important writers from the United States, Canada, England and Australia.

Organized in eight sections, the book opens with an exploration of the past and future possibilities of anarchism, then moves to consider the "necessity" of the state and bureaucratic organization as well as the meaning of the "anarchist contract." The third of the theoretical sections tackles the hard questions for social anarchists confronting the foundations of libertarian socialist and liberal democratic thought. In part four, the contributors traverse the defining characteristics of the various feminisms moving to a concrete statement about the nature of anarchafeminism. In the fifth section about work, the authors consider the issues of worker's self-management, resistance through the underground economy, as well as the implications of the abolition of work itself. In the final three sections, the anthology addresses the culture of anarchy, self-liberation, and the process for building an anarchist society. The book ends with a set of trenchant observations on the current scene by the editor.

Howard J. Ehrlich is the editor of *Social Anarchism*, the premier English-language magazine of anarchist writing. Trained as a sociologist and social psychologist, Ehrlich directs The Prejudice Institute, a national policy research and educational organization studying group prejudice and ethnoviolence in all of its manifestations. He brings a unique blend of social science, anarchist theorizing and community action to this anthology.

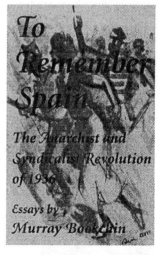

To Remember Spain: The Anarchist And Syndicalist Revolution Of 1936 by Murray Bookchin; ISBN 1 873176 87 2; 80pp two color cover, perfect bound 5-1/2 x 8-1/2; £4.50/$6.00. In these essays, Bookchin places the Spanish Anarchist and anarcho-syndicalist movements of the 1930s in the context of the revolutionary workers' movements of the pre-World War II era. These articles describe, analyze, and evaluate the last of the great proletarian revolutions of the past two centuries. They form indispensable supplements to Bookchin's larger 1977 history, *The Spanish Anarchists: The Heroic Years, 1868–1936* (to be reprinted by AK Press). Read together, these works constitute a highly informative and theoretically significant assessment of the anarchist and anarchosyndicalist movements in Spain. They are invaluable for any reader concerned with the place of the Spanish Revolution in history and with the accomplishments, insights, and failings of the anarchosyndicalist movement.

New Books from AK Press

I Couldn't Paint Golden Angels: Sixty Years of Commonplace Life and Anarchist Agitation by Albert Meltzer. ISBN 1-873176 93 7; 400pp, two color cover, perfect bound 210 x 245 mm; £12.95/$19.95. Albert Meltzer (1920-1996) had been involved actively in class struggles since the age of 15; exceptionally for his generation in having been a convinced Anarchist from the start, without any family background in such activity. *I Couldn't Paint Golden Angels* is a lively, witty account of what he claimed would have been

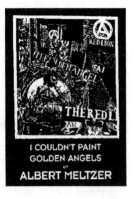

the commonplace life of a worker but for the fact that he spent sixty years in anarchist activism. As a result it is a unique recounting of many struggles otherwise distorted or unrecorded, including the history of the contemporary development of anarchism in Britain and other countries where he was involved, notably Spain.

His story tells of many struggles, including for the first time, the Anglo-Spanish co-operation in the post-War anti-Franco resistance and provides interesting sidelights on, amongst others, the printers' and miners' strikes, fighting Blackshirts and the battle of Cable Street, the so-called Angry Brigade activities, the Anarchist Black Cross, the Cairo Mutiny and wartime German anti-Nazi resistance, the New Left of the 60s, the rise of squatting — and through individuals as varied as Kenyata, Emma Goldman, George Orwell, Guy Aldred and Frank Ridley — all of which have crowded out not only his story, but his life too. *"If I can't have a revolution, what is there to dance about?"* — *Albert Meltzer*

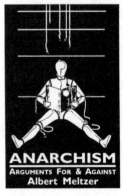

Anarchism: Arguments For and Against by Albert Meltzer. ISBN 1-873176 19-8; 80pp, two color cover, perfect bound 5-1/2 x 8-1/2; £3.50/$5.00 Everything you wanted to know about anarchism, but were afraid to ask. A new revised and updated edition of the definitive pocket primer on anarchism. From the historical background, and justification of anarchism, to the class struggle, organization, and the role of an anarchist in an authoritarian society, this slim volume walks the reader through the salient points, theory and practice, of this much misunderstood and misaligned philosophy. If you're wishing you were better informed, or just mildly curious, this is the place to start.

Friends of AK Press

In the last 12 months, AK Press has published around 15 new titles. In the next 12 months we should be able to publish roughly the same, including new work by Murray Bookchin, CRASS, Daniel Guerin, Noam Chomsky, Jello Biafra, Stewart Home, new audio work from Noam Chomsky, plus more. However, not only are we financially constrained as to what (and how much) we can publish, we already have a huge backlog of excellent material we would like to publish sooner, rather than later. If we had the money, we could easily publish 30 titles in the coming 12 months.

Projects currently being worked on include previously unpublished early anarchist writings by Victor Serge; more work from Noam Chomsky, Murray Bookchin and Stewart Home; Raoul Vaneigem on the surrealists; a new anthology of computer hacking and hacker culture; a short history of British Fascism; the collected writings of Guy Aldred; a new anthology of cutting edge radical fiction and poetry; new work from Freddie Baer; an updated reprint of *The Floodgates of Anarchy*; the autobiography and political writings of former Black Panther and class war prisoner Lorenzo Kom'boa Ervin, and much, much more. As well as working on the new AK Press Audio series, we are also working to set up a new pamphlet series, both to reprint long neglected classics and to present new material in a cheap, accessible format.

Friends of AK Press is a way in which you can directly help us try to realize many more such projects, much faster. Friends pay a minimum of $15/£10 per month into our AK Press account. All moneys received go directly into our publishing. In return, Friends receive (for the duration of their membership), automatically, as and when they appear, one copy free of every new AK Press title. Secondly, they are also entitled to 10 percent discount on everything featured in the current AK Distribution mail-order catalog (upwards of 3,000 titles), on any and every order. Friends, if they wish, can be acknowledged as a Friend in all new AK Press titles.

To find out more on how to contribute to Friends of AK Press, and for a Friends order form, please do write to:

AK Press
PO Box 40682
San Francisco, CA
94140-0682

AK Press
P.O. Box 12766
Edinburgh, Scotland
EH8 9YE